THE CODE CALM MINDSET

Mental Toughness Skills for Nurses in Medical Emergencies

Michael J. Asken & Kimberly I. McMillen

Copyright: 2024

by

Michael J. Asken, MA, PHD

Kimberly McMillen, BS, RN, BSN

This work is subject to full copyright protection. No part of this work may be copied, altered, stored in a retrieval system, transmitted, printed, reproduced, or distributed in any manner whatsoever without the written consent of the authors.

Permissions And Orders May Be Addressed To:

Michael J. Asken, MA, Ph.D.

Kimberly I. McMillen, BS, RN, BSN

PO Box 1065

Camp Hill, PA 17001

dxrxtx@aol.com

Information and data found in this work is believed to be accurate, although it may not be fully representative of all information available in a given area or on a given topic. It is the responsibility of the reader to verify accuracy and assure the validity, the safety, appropriateness and, the liability for any personal or professional use. The information is for instructional purposes only. The techniques described herein are based on both empirical research and experience. Their use does not necessarily provide a guarantee of performance enhancement or safety and no liability is assumed by the authors for their use. Expert guidance is always recommended.

The information contained herein is the work of the authors and does not necessarily represent the official opinions, positions or practices of their associated organization.

Acknowledgments

Although I probably didn't realize it at the time, my mother, an ICU nurse, my grandmother, a surgical nurse, and my father, a physician, were illuminating a path for me into the professionalism and caring of nursing. They showed me, by example, the nobility of being a nurse. Thank you. I also need to express my appreciation to my mentors and nursing colleagues who did and do guide my continuing professional journey. I certainly want to express immeasurable gratitude to my siblings who sustain my commitment to nursing through their own achievements in health care. And to my son, Dylan, you are the reason for trying to make others' lives better and the world a better place for you.

K.I.M.

Baltimore, MD

August 2023

Despite the iconic American image of the lone hero, no one achieves much without the help, guidance and the involvement of others. In addition, if one lives long enough, that list becomes gratefully quite long. So, I will not here attempt to thank all those who have made significant contributions, but gratitude is expressed to my multiple outstanding nursing colleagues from Polyclinic Medical Center and UPMC Pinnacle Hospitals; Harold Yang, MD, PHD; John Goldman, MD; Scott Owens, MD; Danielle Ladie, MD, MPH; and Laurie Schwing, MLS. While they represent the inspirations of the past and present, I must acknowledge those who continue to inspire my future. They are my family: Renie, Kimmie, Dylan, Kaitlyn, Tristen, Jamie, Shay, Cameron, Rylee, Breton and Erin; all of whom have amazed me and continue to do so.

-MJA

Harrisburg, PA 2023

On a regular basis, healthcare professionals are faced with problems that are sudden, unexpected, and potentially threaten a patient's life. These problems don't leave much time for in-depth reflection but demand thoughtful action despite the need for swift decisions. This, as most of us know only too well, is far easier said than done (St. Pierre et al. 2011).

Table of Contents

Foreword i

Preface iii

Introduction 1

I.   Performance Diagnostics:
Your Mental Toughness Psychological Skills Profile 23

II.   Fit for Duty:
Physical Conditioning and Performance 47

III. Mental Lights and Sirens:
Sympathetic Reactions and Performance 64

IV. Mental Alarms:
Stress, Fear, and Performance 84

V. Mental Valium:
Sympathetic Modulation and Performance 127

VI. Mental Scopes:
Concentration Skills and Performance 166

VII. Mental Scans:
Performance Enhancing Mental Imagery & Performance 193

VIII. Mental Prescriptions:
Step-Up, Self-Talk and Performance 238

IX. Mental Ablations:
Negative Thought Stopping and Performance 260

X. Mental Clinical Pathways:
Attitude, Affirmations & Performance 270

Apendix 1 276

References 277

Photo Credits 301

About the Authors 302

Foreword

I am writing this foreword because Kim, my co-author, is a nurse and, with humility, felt it was not right for her to trumpet some observations I can make. Rest assured that Kim has her opinions (strong) and commitment (unwavering) to her nursing and healthcare colleagues. Thank you, Kim, for letting me kick this off.

In these days of full transparency, I should tell you that my wife is a nurse, my two daughters are nurses, my mother-in-law was a nurse, as was her sister. Altogether, this represents experience in ICU, School, Cardiology, High-Risk OB, Surgery, and Administration. This may help explain why a psychologist is involved in writing a book about nursing performance. I had little choice but to learn and respect what nurses do and who they are. And those lessons, both personal and professional, have been borne out, and continue to be demonstrated to me, on a daily basis.

To be trite, nurses are truly the 'glue' that cements the quality and success of patient care. And while the public rightly admires the knowledge and compassion nurses consistently display, they stand in awe of what nurses, and all healthcare providers, do in medical emergencies. Though hyped and dramatized on television, the actions in life and death crises are noble and can approach the miraculous. However, I have also learned that nurses are human and, as such, vary in their skills and response in crisis situations. I have been lucky enough to work with professionals in other HERO, high-expectation, and risk occupations; police, fire, and the military. Here, too, I learned that crisis response can vary. At a time when performance needs to be unhesitating and optimal, it may not be.

But I also learned that the issue is rarely motivation; commitment to help is always a cornerstone. It is the training, understanding and use of the psychological skills that allow the effective and maximal application of knowledge and technical skills which is highly variable and often totally lacking. So, the final thing I learned from my experiences is that psychological performance skills, mental toughness and mindset can be trained and enhanced. And that is why I am so pleased to be part of this book, with its goal to gather disparate knowledge on psychologically maximizing human performance and begin to consolidate it for the benefit of the often superhero nurses and their patients.

Michael J. Asken, MA, PhD

Preface

As a nurse with twenty-nine years of experience, I found The *Code Calm Mindset* to be thought-provoking and a valuable needed resource for nurses caring for patients in all areas of healthcare.

Have you ever been in an emergency where your heart is beating out of your chest, your palms get sweaty, or you just cannot think fast enough? Psychologist Michael Asken and Nurse Kimberly McMillen have provided strategies to help you and all nurses cope with unforeseen medical emergencies while providing a roadmap for ensuring that you remain sharp and at the top of your game when it comes to providing care in high stress and all situations.

Nursing is a profession that requires focused and precise execution of live saving interventions on a daily basis. A rather "normal" and quiet day can turn in to a high-pressured crisis with little to no warning. Nurses need to not only be prepared mentally and physically to respond quickly, but need to be able to respond with optimal performance. Our training prepares us with the techniques to save lives, but not often the skills to confidently and smoothly apply and execute them in a crisis. The **Code Calm Mindset** fills that need.

The state of mind where nurses are prepared for any situation at any given moment to respond in a calm and focused manner is what Asken and McMillen explore in describing mental toughness for medical emergencies. The Mental Toughness Psychological Skills profile (MTPSP) provided in the book will help nurses determine and understand the mental toughness skills they may already have, but which can be strengthened, as well as, highlighting skills to be developed.

The **Code Calm Mindset** provides the concepts and psychological skills for performance enhancement in an easy to understand and practical manner. The authors have done an excellent job providing real life examples from nursing and other mission-critical professions, using relatable analogies that allow nurses to readily implement training techniques and psychological performance skills. Read and enjoy **The Code Calm Mindset** to add a whole new dimension to your care. It will help you and our nursing colleagues understand and use these skills to provide optimal care while managing emergent situations.

-Lisa Swenson MS, BSN, RN, ONC

Introduction

Nurse's motto: 'Every day is one more accomplishment."

- Karen Carlson

Long before you and your nursing colleagues were recognized as heroes for your courageous care during the Covid-19 pandemic, you were part of a HERO profession. HERO (High Expectation and Risk Occupation) is an acronym for those individuals who function where there are the highest expectations of their performance; there is risk to those for whom they care; and sometimes there is risk to themselves.

You provide your heroic care on a daily basis in diverse settings. From the intensity of the ICU, the intermittent chaos of the ED, the careful monitoring of the Medsurg unit, the usual joy, but sometime sorrow, of the OB service, the needs of a child and family on the Peds floor to the humane comfort of Palliative Care, you are challenged to meet the highest expectations of patients, families, physicians, colleagues, supervisors, Systems and yourself.

It is not surprising, then, that you and your colleagues experience stress and burnout. The causes and possible solutions for this unfair side-effect of your skilled and compassionate work are now well recognized and discussed (Bakhamis et al., 2019). There is another source of stress, however, which while recognized, is not addressed as well as it might and should be. This is the stress of the medical emergency, the hallmark of which is the "code" or cardio-pulmonary resuscitation.

While it is the emergency department or critical care unit that may leap to your mind as the typical venues for urgent action, you know that emergencies happen on any floor or service. Life-threatening emergencies occur on the medical floors with the appearance of ventricular tachycardia, in the OR when a patient on the table deteriorates, on the OB service when the most anticipated event in a couple's life presents critical complications, or the pediatric unit where crises involve fearful, protective parents. Nursing students are also often witness to, if not participants in, all of these situations as they contemplate their career choice and decide to seek or avoid such events.

Maybe you considered working in a more tranquil and predictable setting like an office-based practice, but even this may not guarantee insulation from an unexpected emergency and its stress. A common example is the patient who comes to the office complaining of "heartburn" which is really an evolving myocardial infarction.

Then there are situations outside of the office or hospital that call for emergent action. A jellyfish sting while on vacation at the beach, an ankle fracture on a mountain trail, a guest that faints at a social gathering or sporting event, injuries at a motor vehicle accident that you confront on the way home, or even delivering an ill-timed baby are all possibilities as suggested and addressed by Goodspeed & Lee (2007) in their excellent book *What If?*

If there is no doctor 'in the house,' or even if there is, you may become the point person for the crisis. Further, depending on where you are in your career, a medical crisis may occur after your skills for direct action have been dormant for many years or before you have experienced many codes. The expectation for smooth expert action will be high from others, but more importantly from yourself, for that's how nurses are wired.

This constellation of social and psychological expectations assures that administering emergency medical care to a patient who would otherwise die is a very stressful situation for all involved. 'Coding' a patient may actually be frightening to many.

This has been well-recognized among physicians for some time. An early study by Capelle & Paul (1996) found that 79% of residents surveyed reported that 'codes scare me.' In a different study, internal medicine residents were asked to rate their own anxiety about participating in a code (cardiopulmonary resuscitation) using a validated and commonly used research anxiety scale (Asken et al., 2001). The mean anxiety rating reported by the residents was 52.55, far above that of psychiatric patients hospitalized for anxiety (47.74) or hospitalized medical-surgical patients (42.68). A more recent evaluation of first-year residents across multiple specialties found that anticipatory anxiety about participation in codes is still prevalent (Asken et al., 2020). Clearly, many doctors experience high stress in life-threatening situations.

What about nurses? If you talk with your colleagues and they are open with you, it is highly likely they will confide that emergencies create anxiety for them. While it appears this issue is less researched in nursing, the evidence supports similar stresses. Ranse (2008) evaluated graduate registered nurses who had participated in hospital resuscitations in the non-critical care environment. Albeit these nurses were inexperienced in emergency situations, the study found the participants to be 'indecisive,' 'unsure of their decisions' and "unsure of their roles" in the resuscitation event.

Makinnen et al. (2009) reported in their survey that 64% of nurses reported hesitation to perform defibrillation due to anxiety. They concluded that CPR training should a focus on reducing the anxiety which inhibits action. More recent literature suggests that nurses associate performing CPR with stress and look to simulation training to reduce code-related anxiety; however, despite being CPR-trained, many nurses believe their performance to be insufficient (Sok et al. 2020). Clearly, these attitudes may affect the quality of the emergency care provided. Hesitation and anxiety are not acceptable options when you are in this role.

Won't experience lessen my stress in emergencies?

Patricia Hart and her colleagues (2014) suggested that central to developing resilience in nurses is for them to "toughen up" which occurs as the result of experience. As you gain experience with emergency situations, you will no doubt gain confidence. However, the stress of such crises may not simply be the result of being a novice. Experience can, but does not necessarily, prevent performance stress. As one experienced physician reflected:

Over the years, my trepidation at being faced with novel critical-care situations has lessened, but I have to admit my heart still races during 'codes' (Asken, 2022).

Further, research in other areas of mission-critical human performance has shown that experience by itself is not a guaranteed stress buffer. A study done on Navy explosive ordinance disposal technicians, EODs or 'bomb squads,' showed that, while experienced personnel were clearly less stressed than novices during routine and familiar scenarios, any advantage disappeared when confronted with an unexpected and unfamiliar happening (Spierer et al., 2009).

A study of anesthesia residents and physicians (Krage et al., 2014) found that external distractors markedly reduced the quality of cardiopulmonary resuscitation efforts during simulation, regardless of individual experience. The authors recommended 'all team members, including senior healthcare providers,' should have training to improve performance under stressful conditions. Direct psychological skills training can develop confidence and have this confidence occur more quickly than simple accrual of 'experience' garnered from participation in many emergency situations. Experience takes time and assumes successful experiences. Emergencies may not wait and may not be successful.

Won't ACLS and simulation training lessen my stress in emergencies?

You have probably been trained in providing emergency care by lectures and simulation with sophisticated and specifically designed mannequins. These approaches are effective, but what all these strategies lack is direct psychological skills training designed to reduce anxiety and enhance confidence and performance. This may be especially crucial early in a nursing career. As noted, concerns have been raised that even simulation by itself may not be effective in reducing anxiety (Makinnen et al., 2009, Sok, et al. 2020). Access to variable or insufficient simulation experiences can be a problem. And if created and delivered poorly, simulation can create 'training scars' or even greater anxiety that will be difficult to overcome.

Two Questions for You and Your Colleagues

Let us ask you this question: What percentage of success in emergency medical situations do you think is due to your technical skills…and what percentage is due to your psychological skills?

Technical skills are actions like starting IVs, assisting with intubation, placing central lines and defibrillating; psychological skills refer to intellectual and emotional capacities like conceptualizing the nature of the medical crisis, staying focused, making rapid and correct decisions under stress, not getting angry, and not 'freaking out.' Experience and informal survey indicate that health care providers often consider the importance of technical and psychological skills to be equal and often it is the psychological skills which are given the edge as the prerequisite for successful intervention. Our experience is that successful crisis management is reported to be thirty to ninety percent psychological in nature.

If you think about it, perhaps these estimations are not so surprising. The importance of psychological skills and what is often termed 'mindset' or 'mental toughness' in other areas of elite human performance is well-recognized. An obvious example is in competitive sports. The great New York Yankee Hall of Fame catcher, Yogi Berra said:

"Baseball is 90% mental, and the other half is physical."

While probably a better ballplayer and manager than mathematician, he was trying to emphasize the importance of the 'mental game.'

The same awareness exists in the military, even among the most technologically advanced and elite combat teams. John Maxwell (2001) in his book *The 17 Indisputable Laws of Teamwork* has written about the Navy SEALs:

"The key to the success of the SEALs is their training – the real emphasis of which is not learning about weapons or gaining technical skills; it's about strengthening people…"

Given that psychological performance skills are considered so determinative of effective action, let us ask you the second question: How much time do you spend directly training psychological performance-enhancement techniques to maximize your actions in an emergency? If you are like most health care professionals, and even if you said emergency treatment is fifty to ninety percent dependent on mental skills, the time you spend on psychological training is probably minimal, if any at all.

It is likely that, in your training, you have spent time learning about psychological topics like communication, putting patients at ease, dealing with grieving family members, hostile patients, and the difficulties of shift work. You have probably spent little time being taught or studying psychological performance skills. This type of training is rare, as is even its discussion. In fact, a cursory review of random nursing texts finds that psychosocial topics are discussed at length in sections such as 'The Psychosocial Basis of Nursing Procedures.' But among the collective thousands of pages, nothing is found on psychological skills that enhance performance and minimize stress during emergencies (Perry et al., 2016; Hinkle et al., 2022; Potter et al., 2023).

It seems a little puzzling that psychological performance skills for nurses are generally viewed as so highly important while being so largely ignored in mainstream training programs. One thing is clear, however; this is different from other areas where human performance occurs under pressure. Olympic athletes, firefighters, police, and military personnel can all experience significant demands on their performance. However, especially the mission-critical professions, have now developed programs to integrate psychological performance skills to promote elite performance.

A recent trend has been an increasing emphasis on training mindset or mental toughness and psychological skills in physicians, as well. This is especially true in surgery and emergency medicine (Anton et al., 2017; Lauria et al., 2017; Asken 2020;). While these professionals were once only told to manage their stress (suck it up), or consider that maybe they didn't have the 'right stuff,' there are now efforts to formally train physicians and surgeons to develop the psychological skills to produce maximum performance during high stress situations. 'Get over it' or 'deal with it' has been replaced with training on how to get over it, deal with it…or suck it up.

While nursing has evaluated some general resilience-building programs, usually based on the technique of mindfulness, no comparable comprehensive psychological skills programs for emergency situations appear to exist (Mealer et al, 2014; Mealer et al., 2017; Magtibay et al., 2017). To date, we are aware of no extensive studies that have been done to explore these same effects on nurses in high stress situations. Ranse (2008), in the study on nurse response to resuscitation stress, however, did conclude that:

"Strategies should be implemented to provide non-critical care nurses with the confidence and competence to remain involved in the resuscitation process…"

Nursing articles have alluded to the importance of such skills, however. Richardson (2011) proposes that 'in a profession where an off day can seriously affect a patient's health,' pressure must be handled, and the way to do that is to develop mental toughness. Others (Hart et al., 2014) suggest that strengthening and developing personal resilience is key to a successful nursing career and consists of self-efficacy, coping techniques, feelings of control, and competence. These are skills and characteristics which flow from the performance mindset. While not the only thing, the importance of mental toughness in nursing is being acknowledged (Raso, 2021).

Data and experience that are available present a reasonable educational pathway to bolster nursing training and performance. It is, in fact, the understanding and use of psychological performance skills that promotes what is called mental toughness and which can be defined as:

Possessing, understanding, and being able to utilize a set of psychological skill that allows the effective, and even maximal execution or adaptation and persistence of decision-making and clinical skills learned in training and by experience. Mental toughness expresses itself everyday, as well as in high stress, and critical situations.

It should be clear from this definition that mental toughness is in no way incompatible with clinical sensitivity, empathy or rapport. In fact, mental toughness is likely to enhance these essential aspects of care.

It is accepted that solid psychological preparation can reduce the stress of any situation. An area of stress that is receiving increasing attention related to emergency care is that of post-code emotional reactions. This is especially true in the event of an unsuccessful resuscitation attempt. Post-traumatic stress symptoms and critical incident stress reactions have been recognized and described (Laws, 2001; Lippincott Solutions, 2017, Meekin, Hickman, Douglas, et al., 2017). And while post-code stress seems to receive more attention than in-code performance stress in the nursing literature, the mindset techniques that facilitate performance in critical situations may be helpful in mitigating post-emergency stress reactions, as well (Honig &Sultan, 2004).

So, the integration of a mental toughness psychological skills component with nursing skills training can enhance care and reduce the potential negative impact of emergency stress on performance and outcomes. Feeling maximally prepared and confident that your response was optimal, you can feel good and comfortable about your effort, no matter what the ultimate outcome.

In THE CODE CALM MINDSET, we will provide the concepts and psychological skills for performance enhancement in a practical manner based on research in the field of human performance and our experience. Therefore, while references will be made to the sources of the content provided, it will be done to a much lesser degree than in a typical textbook. The sources and more are contained in the bibliography, and material is used from these individuals with respect and appreciation for the contributions they provide.

There are many good things that you can gain from training in mental toughness and psychological performance skills. First, you will gain a foundation in the psychological performance skills that can promote learning, mastery, and application of your technical and decision-making nursing skills to provide an optimal response to manage emergency situations.

As in all areas of high-level human performance, some of you are already highly adept at such performance skills. You are the individuals we study in order to learn what makes you so effective. But, even model individuals can refine their skills or come to better understand what they are doing, resulting in even more flexibility, effectiveness, and safety in their work and the ability to teach others. If you fall into this category, please use this book as an opportunity to gain insight into why you are so good at what you do and pass it on to a colleague or student. Countless patients will benefit.

There are several additional benefits that you can gain from learning about psychological performance skills. You will be able to better maximize the quality of your diagnostic and clinical skills and overall treatment in all situations, not just those of high stress.

Another benefit will be to enhance your confidence in handling the many different types of situations you face. As noted, experience and success are important factors in the development of confidence. Psychological training can accelerate this process and provide support, especially early in a career where it is often needed (Hart et al., 2014).

Learning about psychological performance skills will help you keep your technical skills fresh (White, 2019). Nurses are well aware of the 'stale beer effect,' the degrading of skill quality due to non-use over time. The fortunate or unfortunate reality is that need for many critical skills, especially by non-emergency/non-critical care nurses, can be very infrequent.

Many times 'use it or lose it' skills are, in fact, lost. When was the last time you were involved with the defibrillation or intubation of a newborn? While specific training approaches help keep skills fresh, psychological skills training can also prevent atrophy or 'rust' and promote retention of these skills.

Finally, psychological performance skills are relevant to all aspects of your life. Although the primary goal is improved emergency response, these are performance enhancement skills that can be used to optimize the performance of any nursing or personal skill. Whether you are interviewing for an advanced position, preparing a presentation, or perfecting a yoga position, these techniques can add an important component to your performance.

Does this stuff really work?

Evidence exists for the effectiveness of the techniques to be discussed. Unfortunately, because of the scarcity of such training in nursing, most of the work detailed has occurred in other, sometimes related, and sometimes unrelated, fields.

For example, related to elemental CPR skills, a form of psychological skills education called stress inoculation training was added to standard CPR training in a study by Starr (1987). He found that lay persons who had stress inoculation training in addition to the standard CPR training were less hesitant to use their skills in a test situation and retained a higher percentage of correct skills over time.

Other evidence comes from the pilot study completed with first-year Internal Medicine residents in a community hospital training program discussed earlier (Asken, Zuniga, & Safaee, 2001). The interns underwent 'Code Cool' training comprised of the elements described above. Data analysis indicated there was a significant change in the expected direction in all analyzed affective measures after Code Cool training. The pre-training mean anxiety score was 52.55, and the post-training mean anxiety score was 38.0.

Converging evidence demonstrates that mental skills training can enhance the quality of surgical performance, as has been shown by success in decreasing the perception of stress, maintaining performance under stressful conditions, enhancing specific skill execution, and increasing the use of mental skills (Anton et al., 2017; Anton et al., 2019; Stefanidis et al., 2017).

The use of the specific psychological performance skill of mental imagery has produced a greater sense of well-being and improved self-confidence in nursing students. (Stephens, 1992).

The concepts and techniques described in The Code Calm Mindset are meant to provide you with a basis for psychological skills for enhanced performance. Our understanding of what leads to optimal performance is ever-changing, and unique situations and circumstance call for unique adaptations of these concepts and techniques. We fully encourage you to adapt this material.

Remember that psychological skills training is not a substitute for practice, experience, and other clinical training. The concepts and techniques of The Code Calm Mindset *are meant to be integrated with other training* to provide a truly comprehensive approach to your preparation and performance, especially in emergency situations.

Practicing your skills is crucial. Psychological skills, just as physical skills, need consistent practice to be optimal. There is often a misconception that because something is 'psychological,' simply hearing about it or talking about it is sufficient for mastery. Nothing could be farther from the truth. We are reminded of the words of a piano virtuoso who said:

If I do not practice one day, I know it. If I do not practice the next, the orchestra knows it. If I do not practice on the third day, the whole world knows it.

It is also well-recognized that each nurse, patient, and nurse-patient encounter, despite some common characteristics, is unique. Therefore, you should evaluate and adapt the information in this book as may be appropriate and comfortable for you.

It is clear that those who choose a career in nursing already possess special character, and it is tested on a daily basis. Whether in routine care or emergency situations, each response provides the opportunity for touching and changing patient lives. It has been said (Unknown, possibly US Marine Corps):

Save one life, and you're a hero, save one hundred lives, and you're a nurse.

It is said (Graham, n.d.) that in a 1926 letter from one great writer to another, Ernest Hemingway penned to F. Scott Fitzgerald that 'guts' or courage was the ability to demonstrate *grace under pressure*.

We hope that The Code Calm Mindset may help you cultivate grace under pressure and do this with great confidence and competence.

———————————————

Throughout this book, the pronoun 'she' and the term "nurse" are used predominantly for two reasons: editorial economy or use by the reference source. It is in no way meant to slight male nurses or other-gendered nurses, or any other medical personnel who practice and provide care with such distinction. Their considerable contributions and excellence are duly noted and appreciated. Further, we want to reiterate that while surgery and emergency medicine are used as a model and point of focus for discussion, the concepts and techniques described are equally applicable to emergency situations in any area of health care and by any provider. The use of non-gender-neutral terms in the quotations is present to preserve the accuracy of the quotation; it is acknowledged that some references may be gender-biased.

I. Performance Diagnostics: Your Mental Toughness Psychological Skills Profile

Not all angels have wings; some have scrubs.

-Medelita

Nurses are well aware that a fundamental requirement for success in treating and caring for a patient is acquiring accurate and useful information. The history and physical are the foundations for diagnosis. Knowing 'what you got' gives direction in knowing where to start and where to go. In the 4th Century B.C., the Roman philosopher Seneca observed:

If a man does not know to what port he is steering, no wind is favorable.

The same is true for successfully learning psychological skills for maximizing your response during an emergency. Knowing 'what YOU got' in terms of personal mental toughness and psychological skills will allow you to efficiently use your time and energy to enhance your clinical skills.

You already have considerable psychological skills, given the work you do. However, completing the Mental Toughness Psychological Skills Profile (MTPSP) will help you to be better aware and to better understand the skills you are already using, as well as how to enhance these even further. It will also introduce you to new skills and highlight areas that need to be strengthened.

Below are a series of statements that comprise the MTPSP. For each statement on the profile, you should indicate how often it is true for you or how often it applies to you. There are no trick questions, and the MTPSP will be most helpful if you are open and honest in responding to the statements. There is no benefit in trying to make yourself 'look good.' It will not be helpful to try to make yourself seem more skillful than you are. You probably wouldn't attempt a 'snow job' with nursing skills training, and you shouldn't do it here, either.

Here's how to complete the MTPSP. For each statement, circle or place an X on the number and descriptor that corresponds best to how often the statement is true for you. The choices are **Almost Always** (True); **Often** (True); **Sometimes** (True); **Seldom** (True); or **Almost Never** (True).

For example, responses from a nurse who feels that question 1 is 'often' true and feels that question 2 is 'sometimes' true would look like this:

1 I can handle a crisis situation.

5	X 4	3	2	1
almost always	often	sometimes	seldom	almost never

2 I get nervous or afraid when in an emergency.

1	2	X 3	4	5
almost always	often	sometimes	seldom	almost never

Now do the same with the full Mental Toughness Psychological Skills Profile.

MENTAL TOUGHNESS PSYCHOLOGICAL SKILLS PROFILE (MTPSP)

1. I can handle a crisis situation.

5	4	3	2	1
almost always	often	sometimes	seldom	almost never

2. I get nervous or afraid when in an emergency.

1	2	3	4	5
almost always	often	sometimes	seldom	almost never

3. I can become distracted and lose my focus in an emergency.

1	2	3	4	5
almost always	often	sometimes	seldom	almost never

4. Even if nervous at the start, I can calm down when reacting in an emergency.

5	4	3	2	1
almost always	often	sometimes	seldom	almost never

5. In preparing to react in an emergency, I can picture myself doing well.

5	4	3	2	1
almost always	often	sometimes	seldom	almost never

6. Goals I've set for myself keep me working hard.

5	4	3	2	1
almost always	often	sometimes	seldom	almost never

7. I am a positive thinker when responding to an emergency.

5	4	3	2	1
almost always	often	sometimes	seldom	almost never

8. I eat at least two good balanced meals per day.

5	4	3	2	1
almost always	often	sometimes	seldom	almost never

9. I can lose my confidence very quickly in an emergency.

1	2	3	4	5
almost always	often	sometimes	seldom	almost never

10. My body feels good, "pumped," and ready to go when faced with an emergency.

5	4	3	2	1
almost always	often	sometimes	seldom	almost never

11. My thinking can get "cloudy" during an emergency.

1	2	3	4	5
almost always	often	sometimes	seldom	almost never

12. Even if I am not "up" to responding in an emergency, I can "psych" myself up.

5	4	3	2	1
almost always	often	sometimes	seldom	almost never

13. I mentally practice my nursing and emergency skills.

5	4	3	2	1
almost always	often	sometimes	seldom	almost never

14. I don't need to be pushed to train and learn more.

5	4	3	2	1
almost always	often	sometimes	seldom	almost never

15. I can become negative about myself when reacting in an emergency.

1	2	3	4	5
almost always	often	sometimes	seldom	almost never

16. I get at least seven hours of sleep every night.

5	4	3	2	1
almost always	often	sometimes	seldom	almost never

17. I'm a mentally tough nurse.

5	4	3	2	1
almost always	often	sometimes	seldom	almost never

18. I get angry or frustrated easily when reacting in an emergency.

1	2	3	4	5
almost always	often	sometimes	seldom	almost never

19. I find myself thinking of past mistakes when reacting to a new emergency.

1	2	3	4	5
almost always	often	sometimes	seldom	almost never

20. I can keep my emotions positive and in control when responding in emergencies.

5	4	3	2	1
almost always	often	sometimes	seldom	almost never

21. Mentally rehearsing my emergency nursing skills is easy for me.

5	4	3	2	1
almost always	often	sometimes	seldom	almost never

22. More training and practice are really not necessary for me.

1	2	3	4	5
almost always	often	sometimes	seldom	almost never

23. I can change negative moods into positive ones by controlling my thinking.

5	4	3	2	1
almost always	often	sometimes	seldom	almost never

24. I rarely or never use cigarettes or other tobacco products.

5	4	3	2	1
almost always	often	sometimes	seldom	almost never

25. I have faith in my ability.

5	4	3	2	1
almost always	often	sometimes	seldom	almost never

26. I wish my body wouldn't get so "revved" up during an emergency.

1	2	3	4	5
almost always	often	sometimes	seldom	almost never

27. My concentration is solid/hard to shake in an emergency.

5	4	3	2	1
almost always	often	sometimes	seldom	almost never

28. I can clear any interfering emotions quickly and refocus on my nursing skills when needed.

5	4	3	2	1
almost always	often	sometimes	seldom	almost never

29. I mentally rehearse responding in difficult situations as a way to practice my nursing skills.

5	4	3	2	1
almost always	often	sometimes	seldom	almost never

30. I'm feeling bored and burned out.

1	2	3	4	5
almost always	often	sometimes	seldom	almost never

31. My superiors and nursing colleagues would say I have a good attitude.

5	4	3	2	1
almost always	often	sometimes	seldom	almost never

32. I use fewer than five alcoholic drinks per week.

5	4	3	2	1
almost always	often	sometimes	seldom	almost never

33. I expect to succeed when responding to a medical emergency.

5	4	3	2	1
almost always	often	sometimes	seldom	almost never

34. I'm afraid "I might lose it" under pressure in an emergency.

1	2	3	4	5
almost always	often	sometimes	seldom	almost never

35. The only thing on my mind when reacting in an emergency is applying my skills in that response.

5	4	3	2	1
almost always	often	sometimes	seldom	almost never

36. If I am too "up" or "wired" during an emergency, I can calm myself down.

5	4	3	2	1
almost always	often	sometimes	seldom	almost never

37. It is hard to get a clear image in my mind of myself reacting to an emergency.

1	2	3	4	5
almost always	often	sometimes	seldom	almost never

38. Doing my job gives me a strong sense of pride and honor.

5	4	3	2	1
almost always	often	sometimes	seldom	almost never

39. I worry a lot when responding to an emergency.

1	2	3	4	5
almost always	often	sometimes	seldom	almost never

40. I limit my intake of "junk food" (doughnuts, chips, etc.).

5	4	3	2	1
almost always	often	sometimes	seldom	almost never

41. I think about screwing up even before starting to react in an emergency.

1	2	3	4	5
almost always	often	sometimes	seldom	almost never

42. I am bothered by things like my heart pounding, hand shaking or "butterflies" in my stomach during emergencies.

1	2	3	4	5
almost always	often	sometimes	seldom	almost never

43. I find myself "hoping" to do well rather than being confident about doing well during medical emergencies.

1	2	3	4	5
almost always	often	sometimes	seldom	almost never

44. "Choking" or "Freezing" at a critical time during an emergency is a worry for me.

1	2	3	4	5
almost always	often	sometimes	seldom	almost never

45. When I mentally rehearse my responding, I can really feel all my senses rather than just "seeing myself" react. (I can see, hear, feel, taste & smell the situation).

5	4	3	2	1
almost always	often	sometimes	seldom	almost never

46. The greater and more difficult the challenge, the better I like it.

5	4	3	2	1
almost always	often	sometimes	seldom	almost never

47. It is hard to clear negative thoughts if they enter my mind.

1	2	3	4	5
almost always	often	sometimes	seldom	almost never

48. I do regular aerobic exercise at least 30 minutes at a time at least three days per week.

5	4	3	2	1
almost always	often	sometimes	seldom	almost never

49. I worry I will face a situation I cannot handle.

1	2	3	4	5
almost always	often	sometimes	seldom	almost never

50. If there were something safe and legal I could "take" to keep myself calm during an emergency, it would really help me.

1	2	3	4	5
almost always	often	sometimes	seldom	almost never

51. During an emergency, my attention is more on my body's feelings than on my skills.

1	2	3	4	5
almost always	often	sometimes	seldom	almost never

52. Just thinking about having to react to a medical emergency makes me nervous.

1	2	3	4	5
almost always	often	sometimes	seldom	almost never

53. If I mentally rehearse my emergency skills, I see it like a movie of myself ; it's like watching myself respond, rather than feeling like being in the scene.

1	2	3	4	5
almost always	often	sometimes	seldom	almost never

54. I doubt if I really want to do this job.

1	2	3	4	5
almost always	often	sometimes	seldom	almost never

55. Making a mistake distracts me from going on to complete the emergency response confidently or effectively.

1	2	3	4	5
almost always	often	sometimes	seldom	almost never

56. I drink more than three cups or glasses of caffeinated beverages (coffee, iced tea, coke, etc.) per day.

1	2	3	4	5
almost always	often	sometimes	seldom	almost never

Now that you have completed the MTPSP, you can score your results. If you look at the Mental Toughness Psychological Skills Profile Scoring Sheet, you will see that there are eight categories with numbers below them. These numbers refer to the numbers of the statements you just completed. Go back and transfer the number that indicated your level of agreement with a specific statement to the space next to the same number as the question on the scoring sheet.

For example, if, for question one, you circled or placed an X on 'often,' you should write the number 4 in the space for question '1' under the category of *Confidence*. If you circled or placed an X at 'sometimes' for question two, you should write the number '3' in the space for question two under the category of *Physical Arousal*. Continue to do this for the rest of the statements, transferring the number representing your level of agreement with the statement to the corresponding space on the scoring sheet.

After you have done this, you should add up the numbers for each category, and you will have your total score for each category. You can now graph these scores on the Mental Toughness Psychological Skills Profile to get a visual representation of your skill profile

Mental Toughness Psychological Skills Profile Scoring Sheet

Confidence	Sympathetic Arousal	Attention Control	Sympathetic Control	Imagery Use	Commitment	Self-Talk Use	Physical Condition
1. ___	2. ___	3. ___	4. ___	5. ___	6. ___	7. ___	8. ___
9. ___	10. ___	11. ___	12. ___	13. ___	14. ___	15. ___	16. ___
17. ___	18. ___	19. ___	20. ___	21. ___	22. ___	23. ___	24. ___
25. ___	26. ___	27. ___	28. ___	29. ___	30. ___	31. ___	32. ___
33. ___	34. ___	35. ___	36. ___	37. ___	38. ___	39. ___	40. ___
41. ___	42. ___	43. ___	44. ___	45. ___	46. ___	47. ___	48. ___
49. ___	50. ___	51. ___	52. ___	53. ___	54. ___	55. ___	56. ___
T= ___	T= ___	T= ___	T= ___	T= ___	T= ___	T= ___	T= ___

Mental Toughness Psychological Skills Profile

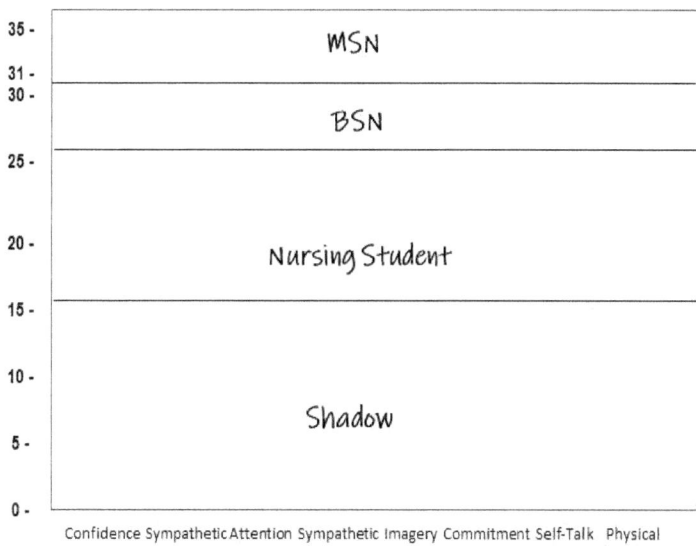

Here is an example of what a MTPSP might look like. What it means and what your profile means is discussed below.

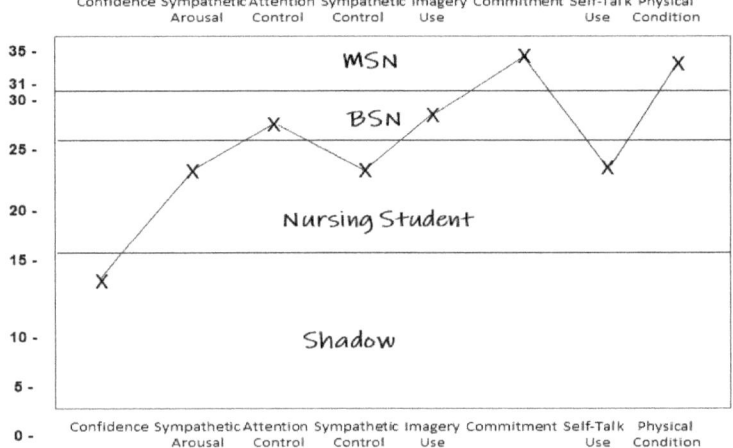

What does your MTPSP mean? You will understand this much better after you have read this book and become more familiar with the psychological aspects of performance. However, a brief description as an introduction is as follows:

Confidence describes the degree of faith you have in your ability to respond effectively during a medical emergency. The category of *Sympathetic Arousal* represents how physically activated or 'pumped-up' you may be during a call – the degree of 'adrenaline rush' you feel. Higher scores here suggest sympathetic arousal, but that which is not problematic. *Attention Control* describes how well you feel you can stay focused during a medical emergency. *Sympathetic Modulation* reflects the degree to which you can control the effects of the adrenaline rush so that they do not interfere with your performance during an emergency. *Imagery Use* describes the degree to which you can use mental imagery or mental rehearsal to imagine yourself responding to various aspects of an emergency as a means of preparation for the response. *Commitment* refers to your degree of satisfaction and positive involvement with your work as a nurse. *Self-Talk* is related to a specific psychological performance factor that affects how your thinking during an emergency influences your performance. Finally, since the mind and body are connected, the last category is a measure of your behaviors that promote optimal *Physical Condition*.

On the graph, the higher your score, the stronger is your psychological skill in that area. Specifically, scores in the range of 31-35 are highly positive and suggest that you are 'a master's nurse' in those skills. A score in the range of 25 to 30 suggests being a 'graduate nurse,' a great foundation for the skill in that area. Scores in the range of 15 to 24 are ok, but you're like a "nursing student" with much to learn. This range of scores suggests that improvement in these areas would be beneficial. If there is a score of 14 or less, the skill needs a lot of improvement, and you are like an enthusiastic volunteer shadowing/following experienced nurses around to begin your education.

Whatever your level on a given psychological skill, The Code Calm Mindset can help you enhance your performance. A very low score on a skill suggests an opportunity to possibly add a whole new dimension to your nursing skills. Even if you are at the 'graduate level,' this manual can help you understand your skill better, refine it, and use it more effectively.

At this point, we want to issue a challenge. The challenge is to be the best nurse you can be and to be open to learning anything that improves the quality of your skills. Although some psychological performance techniques may seem odd or uncomfortable at first, the challenge is to not automatically dismiss them but consider possible use or adaptation.

And if you don't accept the challenge for yourself, we challenge you to maximize your skills for the patients you care for in the emergent and difficult situations in which you work. Finally, we challenge you to be your best for the people who are close to you, proud of you, and support the difficult but crucial work you do.

II. Fit for Duty: Physical Conditioning and Performance

Life is not about how fast you run or how high you climb but how well you bounce.

-Scrubsmag.com

It may seem odd to find a discussion on physical conditioning in a book about psychological skills. However, it should not require much consideration to recognize why this is important. As his career matured, tennis great Jimmy Connors stressed the importance of physical conditioning:

People say I am still around because I have a lot of heart, but I know all the heart in the world couldn't have helped me if I wasn't physically fit.

It is a major focus of this book to describe how the mind and body interact and how they need to function in harmony for optimal nursing emergency performance. True confidence and competence are a combination of physical and mental excellence. There are many issues with maintaining optimal physical status. However, we will comment briefly here on only two areas: exercise and sleep.

Exercise and Physical Conditioning

Physical Impact

The importance of physical conditioning is clear when we acknowledge that emergency medical situations are intense physical and psychological experiences. They are unique in that physical and psychological intensity can initiate immediately, often without warning or preparation. Outside of law enforcement and military operations, few other endeavors expose individuals to this type of immediate assault on their normal physiologic functions.

The evidence is now abundant that exercise produces important physical benefits. We are sure you are well aware of the positive effects of exercise, especially on cardiovascular conditioning. It can reduce resting heart rate and blood pressure and can improve the capacity and efficiency of the heart under stressful conditions. In well-conditioned individuals, the heart rate returns to resting levels more quickly when physical demands are complete.

A highly relevant and instructive study is that of Barnard and his colleagues (1973). They subjected young, healthy men to unexpected, sudden, and strenuous activity (akin to that which might occur when you are summoned emergently to a patient's room and have to sprint down a hallway or maybe even up some stairs with the anticipation of crisis). They monitored their cardiac responses both when they could 'warm up' and also when they could not warm up before the sudden exercise.

Even though the participants were young and healthy, over half showed cardiac changes indicating momentary ischemia with the start of sudden exercise when they did not warm up. However, when they first warmed up, none of the participants showed evidence of any ischemia. While brief decreases in blood flow *may* be handled adequately by young, healthy individuals, the implications could be quite different for the older, perhaps less well-conditioned nurse.

Fitness in the form of strength is often underemphasized relative to aerobic fitness in nursing, but is no less important in medical emergencies. Moving, rolling, and lifting patients is easier with functional strength and less likely to result in injury. Low back pain is a common patient complaint and is no less so in nurses. The frequency of low back pain complaints in nurses ranges from 40% to over 97% (Tosunoz & Oztunc, 2017). Restraining a combative or delirious patient requires strength for effectiveness and your own protection.

Your level of fitness may also affect the quality of care provided. Research has demonstrated that the quality of chest compressions in cardiopulmonary resuscitation decreases quickly due to fatigue. Ochoa et al., (1998) studied ICU and ED staff and found such decreases during CPR. Correct compression performance fell to 79.7% in the first minute; 24.9% in the second minute; 18.0% in the third minute; and 17.7% in the fourth minute. However, the staff was not aware of these decrements in the quality of their efforts.

Baubin and colleagues (1996) looked at the same issue in professional rescuers. The duration of CPR was affected by the method and the individual's work capacity. The authors suggested it is important to improve work capacity through aerobic training in providers.

Psychological Impact

Research is now also very clear that exercise and physical conditioning is associated with positive psychological benefits. It can reduce feelings of depression and anxiety and increase your self-esteem. Regular exercise promotes the release of endorphins, which are associated with improved mood and pain tolerance.

When you are not fit, you have greater sympathetic arousal; when you are well-conditioned, you have a decreased physiological response to stressors. The negative effect of sympathetic arousal on precision skills will be discussed shortly. Overall, with good conditioning, your stress tolerance will be greater; you will demonstrate a more stable mood and show clearer mental functioning under stress.

To summarize, the effects of physical fitness relevant to emergency medical situations include:

- Increased endurance
- Increased physical resistance to stressors
- Increased tolerance of discomfort
- Enhanced mental functioning under stress
- Enhanced and more stable mood

As a side note, the concept of *functional fitness* has become common in firefighting, law enforcement, and military circles. This has also been called the Law of Exercise Specificity (DiNasio, 2006), which emphasizes the importance of designing your exercise program so there is a similarity between the exercises in your program and the physical exertion required by your work.

The United States Marine Corps has adopted a 'functional fitness' model for all of its members. And they differentiate between being 'physically fit' and the higher level of being 'combat fit.' Does your exercise program condition you to bend, lift, stretch, and reach as your job often requires? Does it challenge you to reach a level of 'combat' fitness for whatever you may encounter?

Why are we spending so much time discussing what may be the obvious need and benefits of exercise? Despite all the clear benefits, research still shows that more than 50% of participants will drop out of their exercise programs by six months (Dishman, 1986; PT Direct, 2023). Starting a program is easy and usually done with enthusiasm, but dropping out is so common that exercise has been called the 'four-day phenomenon.' For many nurses, exercise is also a four-letter word: QUIT.

Good information about exercise engagement among nurses is scarce and incomplete. However, information that does exist from the United Kingdom, suggests that 50% of nurses reported low levels of physical activity. While 21% reported exercising every day, 23% reported never exercising; and about 46% of nurses failed to meet the minimum recommended exercise level of 30 minutes five times per week. Seventy-one percent of nurses say they want to exercise more often (Jinks & Daniels, 2003; Brown, 2006; Blake et al., 2011; Torquati, et al., 2017).

This disappointing finding takes on more meaning when it is recognized that 60% of nurses (in Australia) are overweight, leading researchers to conclude that:

Nurses' poor dietary habits and low levels of physical activity place them at increased risk for chronic disease..."(Torquati et al., 2017)

Another missed opportunity from these findings is that nurses, because of their close relationships with patients, can be a model and "point of reference for healthy behaviors," but research shows nurses often exhibit poor lifestyle behaviors themselves (Blake et al., 2011).

Put It to Rest: Sleep and Sleep Deprivation

This brings us to another essential aspect of optimal physical and mental conditioning: quality sleep. You can do everything right and be extra-healthy in lifestyle aspects such as exercise, nutrition, and hydration, but if you sell yourself short on sleep, you will mute the benefits of all your other hard work and discipline.

There are plenty of people who claim to get by on less than six hours of sleep or less, but this is not recommended, nor the norm and it may well affect performance. Given the opportunity to sleep uninterruptedly, we will return to the genetically programmed number of hours we need for sleep.

So yes, you can deprive yourself of sleep for a while, but it will catch up with you.

What is clear from experience and research in both medical and non-medical settings is that excessive fatigue and sleep deprivation can have deleterious effects in many areas of performance. Documented are declines in speed, if not accuracy, of cognitive processing and slowed decision-making. Perhaps most likely, most common, and most pronounced are dramatic declines in your mood and motivation.

Research by Yoo and his colleagues (2007) explained 'the one-two punch' that lack of sleep delivers to emotional functioning and irritability. They found that two things happen in the brain with sleep deprivation. First, the amygdala, which largely produces emotional reactions, became much more active with being sleep-deprived. And secondly, the connectivity between the amygdala and the pre-frontal cortex, which is involved in reasoning and emotional control, was lessened with sleep deprivation. Increased emotion and decreased emotional control explain a lot of the weird stuff that happens when we are tired.

In general, with increasing sleep deprivation:

- Your mood is negatively affected most quickly and to the greatest degree
- Your cognition and thinking are negatively affected more than motor skills
- Your speed is negatively affected more than accuracy
- Your complex tasks are more negatively affected than simple tasks
- Your new skills are negatively affected more than well-learned skills
- Self-paced tasks are least affected
- The longer the task, the greater the negative effect on it

Research (Greer, 2004) also demonstrated that adequate sleep is critical for learning new skills and information. Sleep, especially REM sleep, allows the brain to move information to and store it in long-term memory.

Just like exercise, however, despite knowing the importance of sleep, desirable levels are often not achieved by nurses. Some research suggests that 56% of nurses working night shifts may be considered sleep-deprived (Johnson et al,

2014). About 40% of nurses report not receiving seven hours of sleep per night more than half the time (Blake et al., 2011).

Other research showed that sleep deprivation is associated with lapses in attention on shift. While most nurses demonstrated only one lapse, ten percent of nurses showed nine or more lapses during the observation period (McCann, 2010). Not surprisingly, sleep deprivation is also associated with more patient care errors (Johnson et al, 2014).

Lack of sleep is a threat to nurse influencing health status and being a risk factor for motor vehicle accidents resulting from drowsy driving (Krischke, 2013).

This book is not meant to be a definitive answer on how to get your necessary hours of sleep. Shift work does not necessarily lend itself to good sleep patterns, and most of us have other commitments like families and community involvements that demand our time when nursing responsibilities do not. However, what is also clear from studies on sleep deprivation is that much of our sleep deprivation is really a matter of choice. The point of this brief discussion is simply to encourage you to consider your sleep habits and how they can be improved.

Good sleep hygiene is essential so that when you do get time to sleep, it's beneficial and productive. Google will give you well over 300,000 hits for 'good sleep hygiene,' so there is plenty of information available.

R&R: An Important and Often Ignored Related Concept

An important concept for maximizing performance which is closely related to adequate sleep, is reset and recovery (R&R). The concept is taken from sports conditioning for athletes (Jensen & Asken, 2021). One of the foundational principles of sports conditioning and training for maximal performance is taking a break from intense training and activity. Without adequate recovery, overtraining can occur, leading to decreased performance, profound fatigue, burnout and staleness, mood changes, irritability, and loss of motivation (Eichner, 1995; Skorski et al., 2019).

Dedicated recovery time has been studied and found to be valuable in military training, as well as, being a successful strategy for women in STEM professions (Martin, 2017;

Pritchard, 2015). The military use of recovery dates back to the Roman legions, where soldiers of higher rank and of aristocratic heritage had a refreshment retreat in their tents which they used when they became tired (Scarborough, 1968).

Related to physical fatigue is mental fatigue or 'central fatigue,' which refers to fatigue of the central nervous system. The need to break from intense attention and concentration is required to avoid exhausting the focus circuits in the brain. Relevant neurotransmitters play essential roles in modulating important brain functions, including motivation, arousal, attention, and motor control (Skorski et al., 2019).

Central recovery, then, is an important concept for maintaining high levels of performance. Central or cognitive recovery periods have been labeled by terms such as mental detachment and may be comprised of rest, social engagement, positive, constructive daydreaming, taking a walk, internet surfing, mindfulness exercises, mental imagery, debriefings, music or visiting restorative environments (Purvis et al., 2010).

The concept of 'micro-breaks' would seem to have value and has been discussed by Bertram (2023). These are brief periods of one to five minutes to reset by whatever method works for you. This has been likened to plugging in a cell phone for ten minutes, which will not restore full capacity, but prevents total depletion and inability to function.

One example of a useful microbreak is some form of breathwork. There are many forms, from four-count breathing to eight-count breathing, but it is suggested that any technique where the exhale is longer than the inhale can aid in reducing sympathetic arousal (Bertram, 2023).

Another simple and accessible technique is called panoramic vision. This is the opposite of a focused vision state, where we spend most of our day looking at screens, monitors, phones, etc. Panoramic vision is looking up for a few minutes and taking in a panorama. It is best done outside or with an outside view of nature, cityscape, or horizons.

A mindfulness exercise is also effective for a physiological and psychological reset. Further, when well-practiced, it allows greater awareness of those internal cues telling us when active recovery is needed.

Especially in nursing and medicine, napping is probably one of the most discussed and effective, yet also minimized and ignored, measures for cognitive performance maximization and fatigue management; not so in sports and other fields.

In 2013 the Boston Red Sox addressed sleep and fatigue concerns by placing a nap room in the clubhouse at the suggestion of their sleep consultant. Not only was it popular with players, the team won the World Series that year and the consultant received his own championship ring (Weisfogel & Ross, 2020). In a 28 million-dollar renovation of the Louisiana State University Football Training facility, special considerations were taken to promote recovery for their student-athletes with the installation of locker seats that convert into sleeping pods to facilitate napping (Naintas, 2019).

Major companies like Google, Uber, Nike, Cisco, Zappos, Huffington Post, Proctor & Gamble, and Ben & Jerry's encourage workplace naps and provide accommodations to do so. Federal agencies like NASA and the FAA have traditionally focused on fatigue effects providing opportunities for rest and restoration of cognitive resources (Alger et al, 2019).

Despite a growing interest in strategic napping and mounting data supporting positive performance effects, a continuing cultural bias against napping exists. This bias which equates naps with sloth, weakness, and poor productivity extends to nursing and stifles the effective and creative use of napping to mitigate a variety of stresses plaguing nursing training and practice (White 2006; Geiger-Brown, et al., 2016).

Studies show that lack of recovery, especially in chronically stressful and challenging situations, leads to burnout and breakdown. It ultimately undermines performance. It has consequences that range from 'muscles to motivation.' (Eichner, 1995; Loehr & Schwartz, 2001). The need for respite over prolonged intervals, such as vacations, is well-recognized, though often not heeded in nursing.

Unfortunately, busy clinical responsibilities, coupled with a strong sense of duty, often cause us to 'grind' through without taking a break. R&R will be discussed later as a way to maximize performance and reset after an unexpected event. For now, suffice it to say that the use of R&R has been under-utilized in medical and nursing care, and calls for greater use and acceptance are occurring (Jensen & Asken, 2021). The sports world is changing and incorporating a multimodal approach to rest and recovery. Perhaps it is time to recognize the need for more frequent reset and recovery periods in nursing education and practice, as well.

Guarding and maintaining sleep is important, especially in our sleep-deprived society. Beyond performance, it is useful to remember Greer's comments (2004) that good sleep may well be an important predictor of lifespan and quality of life; or those of Cornell University sleep researcher Dr. James Maas who said that depriving the brain of sleep:

…makes you clumsy, stupid, and unhealthy.

III. Mental Lights and Sirens: Sympathetic Reactions and Performance

I may be compelled to face danger but never fear it, and while our soldiers can stand and fight, I can stand and feed and nurse them.

– Clara Barton

If you really want to optimize performance in emergencies, it is essential for you to understand and control sympathetic reactions or physiological arousal. Sympathetic arousal is related to the well-known 'fight or flight' response. But a third reaction is to 'freeze' and, although perhaps less talked about, it typically represents a major negative performance reaction in high-stress situations. When faced with a medical emergency, fighting or fleeing may not cross your mind, but then again, maybe nothing crosses your mind, and you do nothing, i.e., the freeze reaction.

The quality of your performance under stress is much the result of adrenaline and other stress chemicals released in your body during high-stress situations. Of the three reactions, 'fighting' in terms of expert and fluid application of appropriate skills is what is desired. Fleeing or freezing are clearly not beneficial in a medical emergency. That being said, you should recognize that sympathetic arousal is not all bad.

Arousal can be physical or psychological, and it's called by different terms, such as 'being up,' 'being pumped,' 'amped,' or 'psyched.' There are two types of arousal, and understanding and managing them can have a significant impact on your response in an emergency situation.

Primary arousal, or *task-relevant arousal*, results from the performance demands of the emergency situation. It should provide the necessary preparatory readiness for you to respond. Increased energy and enhanced alertness are part of this preparatory readiness and primary arousal. It can facilitate your actions during an emergency and help you meet the challenge before you.

Secondary arousal, or *task-irrelevant arousal*, however, results from aspects of the emergency situation unrelated to directly meeting the challenge. It may occur as a result of:

➤ Not feeling ready or prepared

➤ A fear of failing

➤ A fear of looking bad in front of others such a your colleagues, other medical and nursing personnel, the patient/family, etc.

➤ Unknowable and/or uncontrollable circumstances

The problem with task-irrelevant arousal is that it is not skill-focused. Its occurrence and intensity are unpredictable; it is harder to control, and it tends to inhibit effective action in an emergency medical situation. It leads to degradation of performance and bad outcomes.

The Sympathetic Arousal-Performance Relationship

The concept of sympathetic reactions like arousal is important because it directly relates to how well you may function during a medical emergency. There are two theories about the relationship between arousal and quality of performance: Drive Theory and Inverted-U Theory.

Drive Theory

In Drive Theory, the relationship of arousal to performance looks like this:

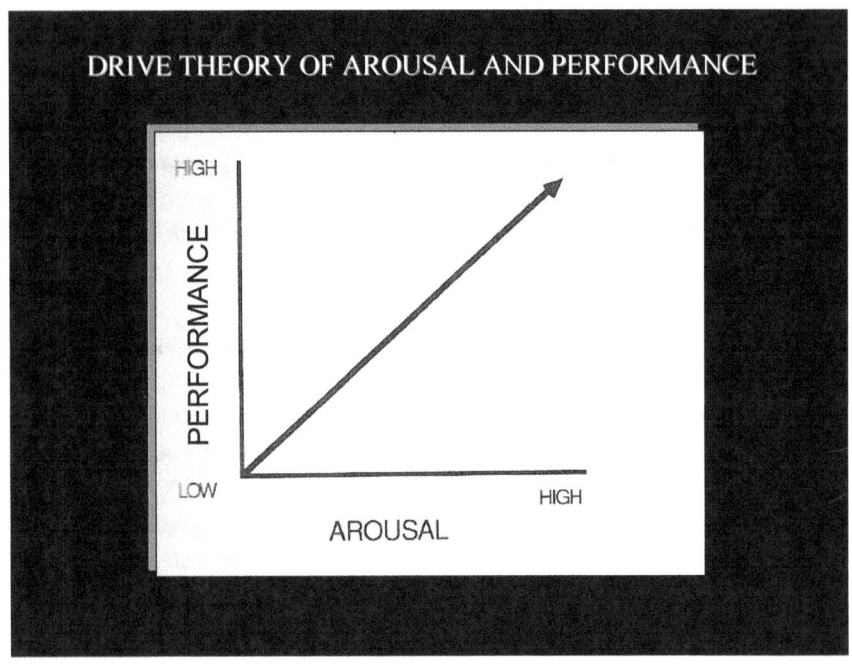

Drive Theory says that when arousal is low, performance will also be low or poor. It says when your arousal is high, your performance will be high or good. In short, the higher your arousal, the better your performance. It suggests that 'more is better,' and arousal can never be too high. A classic example of capitalizing on this theory is football linemen who pound each others' pads and bang helmets to get fired up before the game.

Inverted-U Theory

There is another theory of arousal and performance, however, called the Upside-Down-U or Inverted-U Theory. The formal name is the Yerkes-Dodson Law (from research done on habit formation by the military at the beginning of the last century). It looks like this:

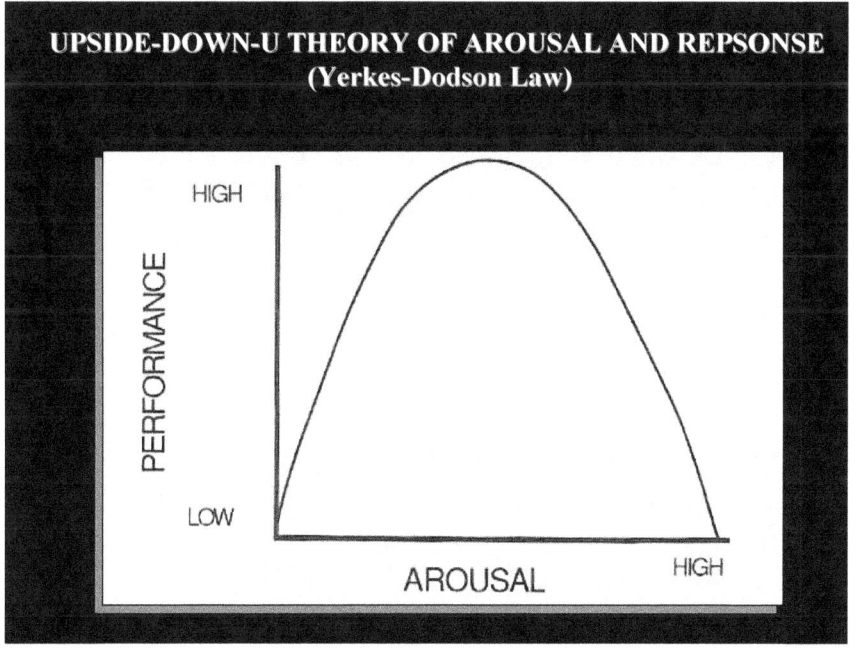

The Inverted-U Theory states that for any skill, task, or situation, you have an 'optimal' level of arousal that leads to peak performance. If there is too little arousal, your performance will be poor. Likewise, if there is too much arousal, your performance will also be poor. Too little arousal fails to make you sharp enough to perform well, while too much arousal becomes distracting and impairs performance.

Which theory do you think is correct?

It appears that most support is for the Inverted-U Theory of arousal and performance. (Know that 'too little arousal' is not the same as being cool under pressure. 'Too little' means there is a lack of sufficient, even minimally necessary physical and psychological readiness to respond to a situation effectively.)

While the Yerkes-Dodson Law suggests that the decline in performance is gradual after sympathetic reactions become extreme, it is worth noting that there is an alternate view with a slightly different characterization (Pargman, 2006). This model suggests that the drop-off in quality of performance after exceeding the ideal level of arousal is not gradual but a dramatic and precipitous 'crash.'

What you should take away from these perspectives is that a sympathetic response to arousal itself is not bad. Sympathetic arousal is an engrained survival response. In fact, we need some degree of arousal to perform at our maximum. Learning how much arousal we need and how to target and control our levels of arousal (modulate) is the key. You don't want to fully quiet all those butterflies in your stomach; that wing-flapping can create valuable positive energy!

In what was truly pioneering work, but today is more of a historical and contextual interest, *Sharpening the Warrior's Edge* author Bruce Siddle (1995) attempted to link this theory and performance to heart rate (HR). He proposed that when HRs approach 115 beats per minute, fine motor skills (like inserting IVs) deteriorate, and when HRs approach 145 beats per minute, complex motor skills (like managing defibrillator patches) deteriorate. He notes that when HRs reach 175 beats per minute or more, there can be, among other problems, a 'catastrophic failure of cognitive processing' (managing defibrillator calculations and settings).

We now know that the HR-performance-quality relationship is not simple or clear. Heart rate *variability* may be a greater influence, and heart rate is not always related to feelings of subjective stress or anxiety. Nonetheless, the concept can serve as a general template for thinking about stress and performance.

It's essential to differentiate between HRs that are elevated because of physical exertion, such as sprinting to a code or from engaging in chest compressions (which is not what we are talking about here), and those elevated due to psychological/emotional stress.

Arousal effects are well-known in sports, with famous pro basketball coach Phil Jackson having remarked:

In a close game, I check my pulse. I know if it gets over one hundred, it's going to affect my thinking.

The medical version of this is the classic adage that 'the first pulse you check in a code is your own.' Whether they knew it or not, the originators of that advice were on to something.

Lima and colleagues (2002) measured stress by HR and blood pressure (BP) in physicians undergoing ACLS training. They found these measures were, indeed, related to stress, and stress had a negative influence on the learning process and efficiency of emergency training.

The Inverted-U effects are not limited to physical skills. Essential to the quality of performance in any situation is what is called 'situational awareness.' This refers to the need for you to be aware of what is happening around you and what it means for current action and for the immediate future. Under stress, you may miss critical changes in patient status or not perceive orders given by the physician-in-charge. Situational awareness is one of the critical *non-technical* skills seen in procedure-heavy specialties such as surgery (Flin, Youngson, et al., 2016).

Situational awareness is also affected by the level of arousal. When there is too much arousal, necessary information cannot be effectively processed; when there is too little arousal, you lose motivation to stay alert. Failure to modulate excessive arousal can interfere with any or all of the essential tasks of situational awareness.

You might fail to see critical cues that are occurring during the crisis or response. You might fail to recognize the importance or meaning of those cues during a crisis or response. Or, you might fail to recognize the next steps required by the critical cues. Situational awareness has been called 'precision in perception' and is critical during an emergency medical situation (Siddle, 2009).

Complicating Factors in the Arousal-Performance Relationship

Like most things, the arousal-performance relationship is not as straightforward as it might seem. There are several factors that complicate the relationship. They are:

- Nature of skill or task

- Complexity of skill or task

- Experience with the skill or task

- Individual characteristics

Different skills or tasks may be performed better with differing levels of arousal. This was first noted in sports (Oxendine, 1970).

Try this out. The following chart displays several sports skills and a scale ranging from 1 to 9. Assume the number 9 represents very high levels of arousal, i.e., you're as pumped as you can get. Assume the number 1 represents very low levels of arousal, i.e., you're almost asleep. Place each skill on the chart based on how much arousal is needed to perform it well.

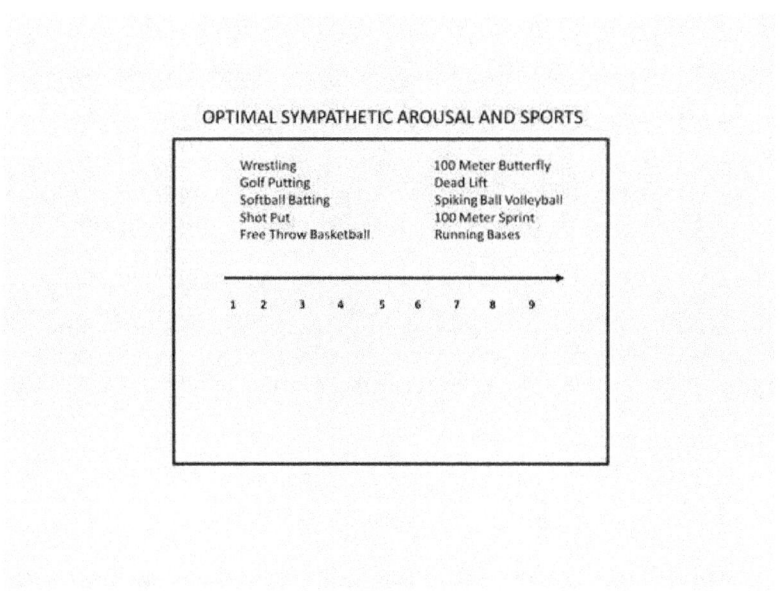

Here are some suggestions for where the skills might be placed in optimal performance.

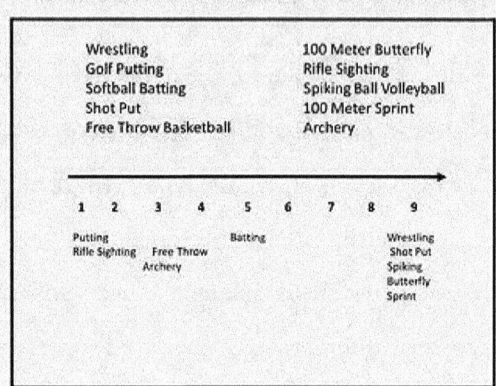

This is not meant to be a rigorous prescription for targeting arousal levels in a sport, but you can see that the arousal level required for quality performance in wrestling or shot-putting is quite different from that which is ideal for putting in golf.

Let's consider the same issue of sympathetic arousal with emergency medical skills. In the following chart, place each of the skills under the number that represents the ideal level of arousal for its optimal performance. Again, the number 9 represents high arousal, and 1 represents low arousal.

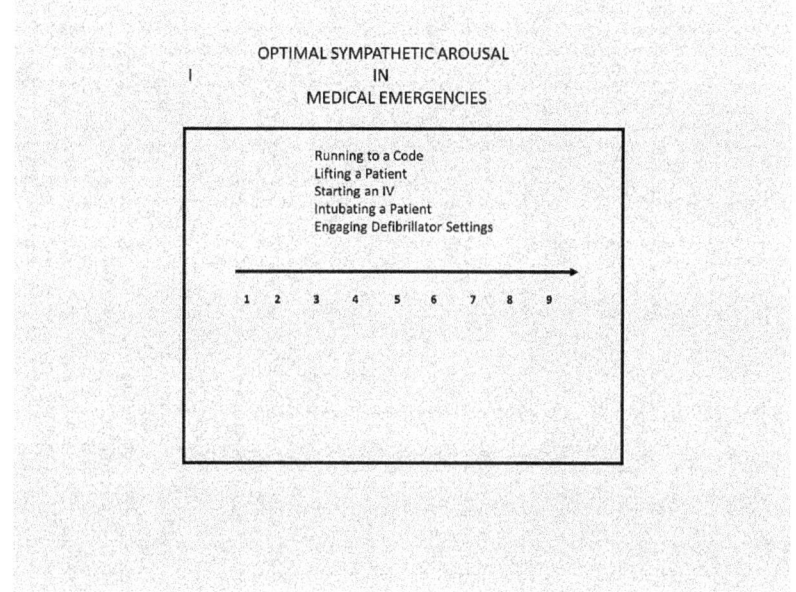

Here are examples of where these skills might be placed.

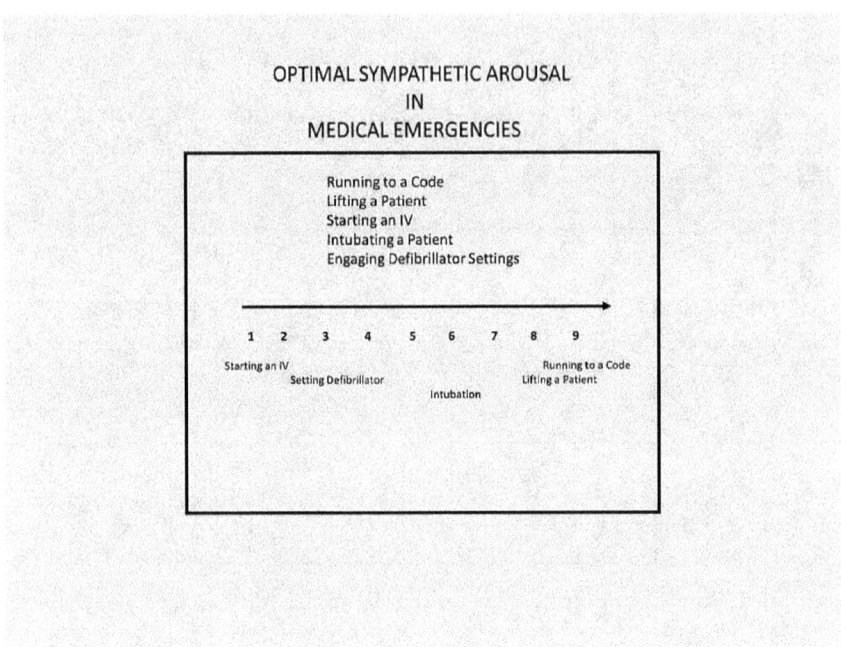

Again, this is not a prescription, and there is no right or wrong response. The point here is to consider that different skills may be performed better at different levels of arousal. Running to a Code (in time!) requires more arousal than starting an IV. The question is whether there is a match between your level of arousal in a given situation and that which maximizes the skill you are applying.

It's interesting to note that most critical skills for medically emergent situations would likely fall on the lower end of the arousal spectrum. This is in spite of the emergency itself tending to generate very high levels of sympathetic arousal. Central lines, difficult intubations, surgical airways, and thoracotomy tubes are all examples. Granted, you may have heard of 'slamming in' a chest tube, but you'll never hear a directive to 'slam in' that central line or ET tube. These things need to be done quickly but with finesse.

The complexity of the skill is another important factor in how levels of arousal affect the quality of performance. Simple tasks can tolerate more arousal than complex ones. This is why football linemen can and need to get pumped up. Without wanting to insult them in any way, the lineman's job of blocking a single player is generally less complex than the job of a quarterback. Quarterbacking requires reading the defense, scanning the field, looking for the receiver, defining the target, making a split-second decision, and throwing the ball with precision, all while the field is in a dynamic state of rapid change. You may or may not be quarterbacking the code, but you need a quarterback's brain.

Another consideration in the relationship between arousal and performance is experience. Skills that have been well-learned (over-learned) allow higher levels of arousal without becoming impaired than newly learned skills. That is why experts may still function in a 'condition black' (really high-stress levels) that would likely be disruptive to someone less skilled and practiced.

Experience engrains a skill so that it is much harder to disrupt it under any condition, including one of stress and arousal. This is the rationale for repetitive training, particularly for high-stress situations. When things go bad, you resort to your training and the neuromuscular connections that have been made, i.e., muscle memory. It has been said: "You don't get smarter in a code." Put another way. It has been observed (Grossman& Christensen, 2008):

You don't rise to the occasion; you sink to your level of training.

When that stressful event happens, and you feel the urge to fight, flee, or freeze, it's your training that will carry the day. Finally, the level of arousal varies by individual, by the uniqueness of every nurse. Some nurses perform better with more sympathetic arousal, while others need to be as relaxed as possible to perform their best. You've likely already seen this in your colleagues. Some look like they just chugged a super-sized Starbucks before they run a code, but it goes off without a hitch. Others appear so mellow they seem to not care. But the results are the same.

Your O-ZONE; What is it?

One of the biggest mistakes that sports coaches, but also nursing faculty, BLS/ACLS trainers, and nurses themselves make is believing that everyone needs the same level of arousal to perform well. This is simply not the case. The key is for you to find your optimal level of sympathetic arousal or what we call your O-ZONE; your *optimal zone of nurtured excellence*, to maximize your performance.

Where do you perform your best? This is what athletes refer to as 'getting psyched-up,' and being 'in the zone.' NASA calls this being in your MAX-Q. Remember, feeling some arousal should be seen/felt as a good thing, as a sign of readiness to respond and perform at your best. Finding your O-ZONE is the key.

Research (Ferrell, 2006) suggests that what athletes call 'being in the zone' is a 'real thing.' There appears to be an actual performance mental zone state, one that is different from other performance states. Using Functional Magnetic Resonance Imaging (FMRI), researchers were able to show differences in brain activation between recall of zone (high level) performance and non-zone (regular) performance. The researchers feel that this initial data support the reality of a "...palpable, yet enigmatic sensation that many athletes refer to as the 'zone' when performing at high levels."

With experience, you will become more aware of your O-ZONE; but you can also help determine it in two ways. Use the chart below to help you assess your O-ZONE levels.

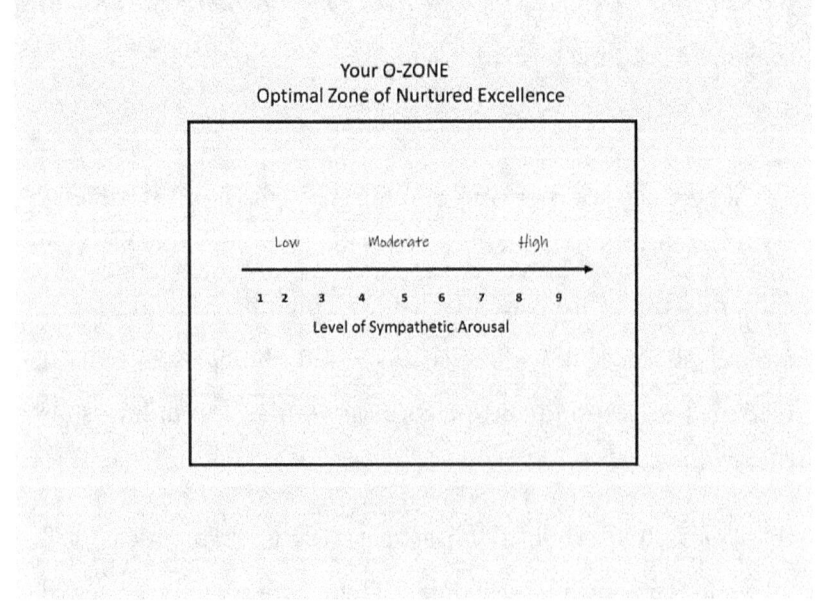

First, think about your most successful medical emergency experiences. These are experiences where you were in the zone and on your game. If you have not yet faced any emergencies, think about other medical, academic, or life challenges in which you performed well. On a scale of one to nine, where one represents being very relaxed, and nine represents being really revved up, how high was your arousal? Then think about a time when you did not perform the way you would have liked or things did not go well. Where was your level of arousal in that situation?

Analyzing the relationship between the quality of personal performance and your level of arousal on past emergencies or challenges may show a consistent pattern indicating what level is associated with your best performance.

There is some suggestion from work in this area (Tennenbaum, et al., 2008) that on a scale of one to nine, optimal performance is most likely to occur in a perceived range of 5.2-6.5. Performance is likely to be decreased with excessive arousal above a rating of 6.8 and insufficient arousal below a rating of 4.0. However, remember that the nature of the task and your nature as an individual are important moderating factors in the arousal–performance relationship.

Another way to help determine your O-ZONE is to do multiple or repeat training simulations in which you perform after getting yourself into different levels of sympathetic arousal: high, low, or in-between. Try out different levels of arousal during training and then consider these questions: At what level did you feel most comfortable? At what level did you do your best? At what level was your thinking the clearest?

As will be discussed later, while adrenaline-related arousal under stress can have life-saving and performance-enhancing effects, it can also degrade performance to dangerous levels. Learning to recognize your optimal performance state, your OZONE, and then using the techniques discussed throughout this book to achieve it can help maximize your performance and your care to the patient.

IV. Mental Alarms:
Stress, Fear, and Performance

Panic plays no part in the training of a nurse.

-Elizabeth Kenny

Performance Stress

Learning the psychological techniques to manage your performance stress not only reduces your discomfort, but can enhance your performance, as well. Somewhat different from life stress or career stress, emergency performance stress can be defined as and can occur any time there is:

> *A perceived imbalance between the demands of the emergency situation and your ability to meet those demands where failure to do so has important consequences to you.*

While this definition is a bit cumbersome, it contains several important components that are necessary to understand performance stress, how it works, and how to control it.

First, stress is very much the result of perception, how you view a situation. In fact, there are three psychological aspects to any medical emergency situation. They are the:

- Objective situation
- Appraisal (perception) of the situation
- Emotional/Behavioral/ Psychological/ Physiological consequences

The objective situation refers to the nature of the medical emergency, the facts of it, something that can be largely agreed upon by everyone. Faced with an objective situation or challenge, you then make an appraisal of the situation and evaluate your ability to deal with it. This leads to a response that has emotional, behavioral, psychological, and physical reactions that affect the quality of your performance.

Where your appraisal/evaluation is such that you feel prepared to act, your stress will be minimal, you will feel confident, and you will be in your O-ZONE. There is a balance between the demands of the situation and your perception of your ability to handle them. However, whenever you feel ill-prepared (by lack of training, experience, information, equipment, back-up, etc.) your stress will increase. Here, there is an imbalance between your perception of your degree of ability and the intensity of the challenge facing you. The specific impact of this stress will be described shortly.

The fact that perception determines your stress level explains why people can have such differing reactions to the same situation. This is most evident between you and your friends who have non-medical jobs. Many people who are quite capable of handling all kinds of stress, from trading stocks to climbing telephone poles, will often tell you there is no way they could handle the stressors of your job. Similarly, you may not be able to handle the stress of their jobs.

More importantly, even within your own profession, there are certain situations that, although stressful, you prefer to handle compared to your colleagues. Dysrhythmias may be your thing…while you dread the overdose patient…while your colleague prefers the high-risk pregnancy. Whatever the circumstances, hopefully, there is congruence between the objective situation and the ability to handle it. However, because perception plays such a large role, some individuals will feel unready to respond when, indeed, they might be very capable. Others may feel very confident when perhaps more reservation is warranted.

This definition of medical emergency stress also points out that stress occurs only when you care about the consequences of not succeeding. If you are indifferent to the situation and outcome (don't give a !@#$%), there is no stress. This, of course, should never be the case as a nurse. When the outcome matters most, and you're invested in doing well, you may be most likely to feel stress. Caring about the outcome and caring for the patient is, of course, is, the foundation of Nursing.

While all medical emergencies can be stressful, some will be situations of high stress. There are specific characteristics of high-stress situations (Driskell, Salas, & Johnston, 2006). These include:

- ➢ There are sudden and unexpected demands that disrupt normal procedures.

> The consequences of poor performance are immediate and severe.

> The task environment is complex and unpredictable.

> You are required to perform multiple tasks under adverse conditions.

High-stress situations occur suddenly and unexpectedly, placing demands on you that were unanticipated (such as expecting a quiet night when, instead, all kinds of stuff hits the fan). Events can unfold quickly, requiring an immediate response. Consequently, normal and routine procedures can be interrupted. Participating in a code with a full bladder or an empty stomach certainly doesn't make the situation easier. It would be nice if patients would only code after dinner and bathroom breaks.

High-stress situations have critical consequences and effects. They demand your full and efficient response. Poor performance, or failure, will have a dire impact during and/or after the response, all of which impacts the patient, yourself, and others.

High-stress situations are typically complex, dynamic, variable, and often unpredictable. Their cause or immediate nature may be unclear. An effective response may be outside of standard operating procedures and require adaptations or creative solutions. Or, your plan disintegrates as new symptoms or problems appear.

High-stress situations typically require you to perform multiple tasks quickly and even simultaneously and/or under adverse conditions. Delay in the arrival of the anesthesiologist, expired medication, and equipment that is missing or not where it should be on the crash cart all increase stress and may demand extra actions on your part. When mentally prepared, you function at an almost automatic level in these complex circumstances.

The physical signs of stress are probably familiar to you. In some circles, they are nicknamed the 'pucker factor,' referring to the sphincter response under stress! They include reactions such as:

- Upset stomach/ butterflies/ nausea
- Increased heart rate

- Increased blood pressure
- Increased respiration rate
- Increased perspiration
- Sweaty palms
- Muscle tightness
- Dizziness
- Bowel/bladder urgency
- Visual changes
- Dry mouth
- Fatigue
- Restlessness
- Chest pain
- Tremors
- Shakes
- Concentration problems
- Word-finding problems

Gonzales (2005) notes that the physical and performance effects of out-of-control stress have been likened to a 'knife fight in a phone booth.' He also extended Plato's analogy of stress as a model of a jockey and racehorse at the starting gate:

The human organism, then, is like a thoroughbred at the gate.

He's a small man, and it's a big horse, and if it decides to get excited in that small metal cage, the jockey is going to get mangled, possibly killed.

So, he takes great care to be gentle. The jockey is the reason, and the horse is emotion…

The jockey is your rational self, and the horse is your emotional self. When under control and in your O-ZONE, your performance is focused, efficient, and maximal. However, if scared and rampaging in the stall, the horse (your emotion) is out of control, and performance is negatively affected. It has been said that unchecked, extreme stress is an *emotional and physical carnivore* (Grossman, 2004).

Amidst all the discussion of the potential negative effects of stress as expressed in what is often called 'the adrenaline dump,' it seems important to re-emphasize that the body's stress response (especially adrenaline release) has positive performance effects, as well. We are all aware of stories of individuals who, in life-threatening situations, have summoned uncommon strength and other life-saving actions. And remember that the performance-arousal curve posits that we need some degree of arousal to perform our best. When arousal is trained and restrained, then stressful conditions become less threatening and more challenging (Ghannam, 2009).

It is the failure to understand, control, and channel the effects of sympathetic physiological arousal (untrained and unrestrained arousal) that can impede your performance and lead to extreme actions that can be problematic. Often this is seen in a rush to action before a clear diagnosis or clear indication for an action is present. The impact of stress on decision-making is discussed later.

Navy Physician Richard Jadick, in his book *On Call in Hell (2007)* about his experiences in Iraq, provides an example of how the effects of stress and adrenaline on thinking can result in a rush to action:

Word came back: wounded Marines. Johns handed off his weapon, grabbed his med bag, and started sprinting the 150 yards to the lead truck. "I wasn't even thinking about it for the first hundred meters," Johns recalls now, "but then it hit me. This is how they initiate ambushes. We're going to get hit right now, and I'm running down the road by myself."

Emergency physician and mountain medicine doctor, Chris Van Tilburg (2007), describes how a rush to action occurs and why it must be controlled:

Spiked with adrenaline, I nearly knock over the forest ranger, who is keeping hikers off the trail. I have room to run. But I force myself to slow down to a fast trot; the last thing I need is to sprain my ankle running up the trail…

In the civilian setting, stress can heighten its own form of 'rescue fever,' leading to failure to thoroughly evaluate a situation before acting. That's why one of the first rules of EMS is to decide, "Is the scene safe?" Most providers want to jump right in, but becoming a casualty yourself isn't the way to do that. Or, it can lead to excessively intense actions which may be inappropriate, intimidating, or disruptive to personal and team performance. It can lead to you figuratively running down the road by yourself.

From a performance perspective, the common physical disruptions of stress include:

- ➢ Choking
- ➢ Freezing
- ➢ Death grip
- ➢ Muscle tension and fatigue
- ➢ Disrupted coordination
- ➢ Blurred vision

Elite performers are well aware of certain physical effects that occur with stress that directly affect the quality of their actions. Choking refers to failing to be able to perform at a critical moment. While it refers to any type of 'failure' response, it comes from the sensation of being unable to breathe or swallow under stress.

So what happens when you 'choke?' Are your skills suddenly and actually gone? It has been explained like this: (Murray quoting Hamblin, 2005):

In reality, athletes do not lose their physical ability, technical skills, and strategic knowledge during a competition. Rather, they lose control of cognitive factors such as the ability to concentrate, focus on relevant cues, engage in positive self-talk, and so forth.

It's reassuring to know that your skills are still there even when you feel like they're not. Just like the Olympic diver doesn't suddenly forget how to do a reverse three-and-a-half somersault off the 10m platform, you haven't forgotten how to start an IV or place defibrillator pads, even if it feels like you did.

The death grip, holding on to something too tightly and longer than needed or desirable, is also a form of choking or freezing. Fluid movement, flexibility, speed, and delicate touch occur most readily when muscles are loose and relaxed. Muscle tension interferes with and degrades these aspects of maximal technique, thereby decreasing coordination.

Further, when muscles are tight, they expend more energy, and fatigue occurs more rapidly.

We will discuss tunnel vision later, but also know that stress can cause a loss of near vision that can make it hard to visually focus or see detail.

The performance effects of stress on human performance have also been described in this manner:

- ➤ Decreased awareness of environmental cues
- ➤ Decreased ability to manage anxiety
- ➤ Decreased tolerance for pain and frustration
- ➤ Decreased ability to deal with errors
- ➤ Decreased efficiency in mental processing
- ➤ Increased mistakes

Decreased awareness of environmental cues means that you become less aware of what is going on around you, what we have discussed as situational awareness. It's often a manifestation of what is called tunnel vision, where your awareness constricts and focuses on a limited area or just one object. It is a loss of situational awareness and often the critical information that you need.

The potential problem with typical reactions like tunnel vision has been well described by Leach in his book Survival Psychology (1994):

Perceptual narrowing appears to be a manifestation of restricted attention. There is a narrowing of awareness coupled with an intensification on only one task. While this intensification enables a person to concentrate on a selected task, there is no guarantee that the task so selected is the most appropriate one in the circumstances. Furthermore, the task can overwhelm the victim, blocking out other, perhaps vital, information needed for effective functioning and limiting the number of alternative responses available…

When your awareness becomes tunneled, you might become more focused and sensitive to signs of anxiety in your body. So instead of being focused on the challenge, you're distracted by butterflies in your stomach, the shakes in your hands, or the need to urinate. You lose your ability to manage or tolerate anxiety, and stress becomes significantly increased.

Stress decreases your tolerance for pain and frustration. Medical emergencies, especially those of a protracted nature, involve discomfort from fatigue and uncomfortable positions. Stress reduces your ability to tolerate these discomforts and increases the chance you will act more quickly and impulsively to reduce your discomfort.

Stress can affect your mental efficiency so that your decisions become less clear and harder to make; mistakes become more frequent. You might have trouble remembering the details or names of the instruments you need. When mistakes occur under stress, we tend to focus on them; it becomes harder to respond and fix them or work around them and recover and move on.

These effects of stress on performance have been called the Sudden Stress Syndrome (Duran and Nasci, 2000), and it has been defined this way:

Physiologic changes that occur as a result of sudden and extreme stress, as well as, the effects the changes can have on your perception and your motor skill performance.

An important part of the Sudden Stress Syndrome is perceptual changes and distortions that occur under stress. Some were mentioned before, but an expanded list of typical perceptual changes in high-stress situations includes:

- Tunnel Vision (Peripheral Narrowing)
- Tunnel Hearing (Auditory Exclusion)
- Intensified Sounds
- Heightened Visual Clarity
- "Automatic Pilot" (action with minimal or no subjectively perceived thinking)
- Time Distortion
- Memory-related Distortions
- Dissociation
- Intrusive Distracting Thoughts
- Temporary Paralysis

The original work on perceptual change in stressful situations was done on police officers (Artwohl & Christiansen, 1997; Artwohl, 2002). More recent work has begun to gather perceptual distortions in firefighters, but also physicians, emergency medicine doctors, and surgeons, when in stressful situations (Nurenberg & Asken, 2015; Levitan et al., Asken et al., 2022).

As the chart below shows, distortions in perception are very frequent across professions in high-stress situations.

Percent of Individuals in Various Professions Experiencing Perceptual Distortions Under Stress

Perceptual Change	Police N=72	Fire N=?	Emergency Medicine N=21	Surgery N=33
Auditory Exclusion	85	89	55	39
Tunnel Vision	82	91	62	39
Auto-Pilot	78	90	76	73
Increased Visual Clarity	65	62	75	32
Time Distortion (Slowed)	63	80	67	58
Memory Distortion	19	74	20	18
Dissociation	50	52	19	27
Intrusive Thoughts	63	47	43	30
Intensified Sounds	17	63	35	33
Temporary Paralysis (Freeze Response)	11 (Artwohl & Christensen 1994)	49 (Asken/Nurenberg 2015)	52 (Levitan, Butler & Asken 2015)	15 (Asken, Owens Tadin 2022)

Recent research by Asken, Forney & Bernal (2023), looked at perceptual changes under the stress of a surgical emergency reported by OR nurses and perioperative personnel. As can been seen in the chart below, perceptual distortion is common in nurses, as well, in high stress situations.

Percent of Nurses and Other OR Staff Having Experienced the Perceptual Distortion at Least Once During a Surgical Emergency
N=165

DIMINISHED SOUND	37
TUNNEL VISION	37
AUTO-PILOT	76
INCREASED VISUAL CLARITY	36
TIME DISTORTION (slow)	65
MEMORY DISTORTION	33
DISSOCIATION	28
INTRUSIVE THOUGHTS	29
INTENSIFIED SOUND	45
TEMPORARY PARALYSIS	27

Auditory exclusion, or tunnel hearing, occurs when we seem to hear only selected words or sounds. It can lead to missing important information to guide emergency actions. It can also lead to team friction because of missing or appearing to ignore input from others.

Sounds may become intensified. Certain sounds may grab your attention and seem particularly loud or clear. The same may occur with your vision; certain objects may stand out and seem brighter and/or sharper than normal.

Automatic pilot means you feel as though you're functioning and responding without needing to think about your actions. This may reflect expertise and confidence, but it may also represent a lack of situational awareness and inflexibility.

Individuals in high-stress situations may experience time distortion. Time usually seems to slow, but it may also seem to speed up.

Memory inconsistencies are quite common in high-stress situations. There may be loss of memory for certain events or actions, or there may be memory distortion. It is not uncommon to believe something occurred in a high-stress situation that in reality, did not.

Dissociation is different from the automatic pilot; it is feeling apart from your actions and the event. It is often described as being 'outside yourself' and perhaps even watching yourself and the event occur.

Finally, temporary paralysis refers to the third common response to stress we mentioned earlier, freezing. This can be a full inability to move or just a feeling that one is slow and ponderous in action. This is illustrated again in the words of Navy physician Lieutenant Commander Jadick as he describes this effect of stress early in his experience in Iraq:

I stepped off the truck and noticed that everything was heavy. Holy f--k, am I even going to make it? Fear is like deep water, slowing every step…

Less dramatic, but much more common is the situation described by Goodspeed and Lee (2007) of (ironically) freezing when being on the 'hot seat' during morning rounds with a demanding attending physician:

It's amazing what can happen when someone is put on the "hot seat." The most outgoing and sociable students can lose the ability to talk. The most knowledgeable can forget answers to basic questions. The most poised can melt in a pool of sweat. Call it stage fright, performance anxiety, or nerves, funny things can happen when you feel exposed in front of a group of people.

It's important to emphasize that while these effects are not infrequent or abnormal, they can profoundly affect the quality of your response in an emergency situation. There are other effects of stress on performance.

One of these is bilateral symmetry which means that what you do on one side of your body, you also do on the other. The term sympathetic contractions and mirror movements have also been used to refer to involuntary contractions that may occur in the muscles of one limb when the muscles in another limb are performing an intended forceful action.

This is related to the Moro reflex seen in infants who, when startled, jerk both hands and legs simultaneously. Under stress, adults can have a similar reaction, as well. Therefore, you must be cautious in situations in which you grab for something or someone with one hand while holding an instrument in your other hand. Reaching to forcefully restrain a patient's arm with one hand while holding something delicate with the other hand is a bad combination. When stressed, you're likely to crush that delicate object to match the force you're using on the other limb. When starting an IV on a combative patient, that delicate object may be the vein you perforate.

A final important effect of stress is a return to not only more simplistic responses, but to those that are most basic, preferred, or dominant for you. The brain requires eight to ten seconds to process each piece of complex and novel information. If there are no immediate or trained responses for the situation, your mind searches for the *"first fix in its library of habits"* (Time, 2005).

An example of this involves a noted psychologist at the University of Wisconsin who, in the past, was asked to help investigate 'unexplained' scuba diving deaths – instances where divers drowned despite having adequate air in their tanks. It turned out that some of these deaths could be explained by the above principle and a return to basic or dominant responses under stress.

The dominant response for human beings when choking or having trouble breathing with something in or something covering their mouths is to (often frantically) remove whatever is in their mouth. The maneuver is effective on land but has the opposite effect underwater when a panicked scuba diver frantically removes their mouthpiece/regulator underwater.

This is why training and practice are so crucial. Navy SEALs undergo 'drown-proofing' where they are repeatedly placed in uncomfortable situations of limited air/oxygen so they can be familiar with the sensations and respond effectively despite the discomfort that would be disorienting and paralyzing to most of us. Such training is needed to override our natural and untrained responses, especially since these are the ones most likely to occur under stress.

What's Happening in Your Brain Under Stress?

The understanding of neuro-performance and the brain comes largely from the work of Nobel-prize-winning psychologist Daniel Kahneman (2013). He posits two systems in the brain related to performance. System 1 is represented in the amygdala, a phylogenetically older part of the brain responsible for threat detection and arousal. It tends to 'assume the worst' in a given situation. System 2 is represented in the frontal lobes, the newest regions of the brain from the perspective of evolution. The frontal lobes are seen as the thinking part of the brain and account for our 'humanness.' The frontal lobes are responsible for what is termed 'executive functions,' higher-order cognitive skills like planning and recognition of consequences.

System 1 and the amygdala provide automatic responses that usually are not in conscious awareness. These are intuitive responses and are characterized by terms like *a gut feeling*, the *"hairs stood up on the back of my neck,"* or *"something ain't right here."*

System 2 and the frontal lobes involve a very much conscious awareness and require significant energy. System 2 also scans for danger, evaluates the System 1 message, and may inhibit action.

A typical illustrative example is if you are walking in a field and suddenly see a three-foot-long black serpentine object, the amygdala will cause you to freeze or jump back, suggesting danger and maybe a snake. The frontal lobes will evaluate all the information you have from the perception and knowledge of snakes and decide if this is truly a threat, a tree branch, or a garden hose.

Another often used and useful analogy is to think of System 1 and the amygdala as a race car and System 2 and the frontal lobes as a pace car which limits the speed of the race car. When someone expresses, "I just acted," "I didn't think about it," or "I just did what I had to do," they are expressing subjective descriptions of System1 functioning. Comments like "Think before you act," "You didn't think it through," or "Measure twice, cut one" represent System 2 frontal lobe functioning.

These distinctions are significant for performance under stress. As can be concluded, System 1 is much more immediate and even impulsive in action, whereas System 2 is much more measured in response. Nursing care usually involves considered actions, but under stress, the two systems function differently.

This is shown in the illustration below, adapted from the work of Dr. Janet Metcalfe at Columbia University.

STRESS AND SYSTEM 1 AND 2 FUNCTIONING

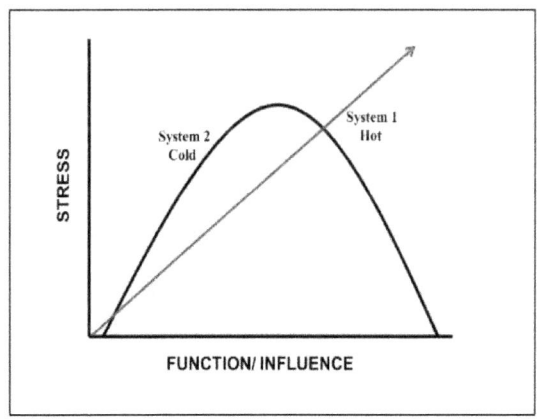

It can be seen in the illustration that System 2 is called the cold system since it is deliberate in nature and follows the familiar upside-down U pattern. Logical (rational?) thinking is enhanced by slight arousal from stress but will lose or cease function when overwhelmed by stress. System 2, however, with its impulsive nature, is called the hot system and continues to gain intensity with stress, especially if System 2 has become dysfunctional and cannot mitigate it. When it is said of a person's irrational and unacceptable behavior, "They just lost it," what is being described is likely this influence of System 1 with a failure of System 2; not a desirable state in nursing and certainly not in an emergency situation.

This description also demonstrates why it is so important to understand the performance effects of stress. Without this knowledge to serve as a foundation for training, nurses may become perplexed and distracted and misinterpret what is happening to them under stress. They may see normal responses as abnormal and feel they are 'losing it.' They may have heard things about how they should or should not respond in a high-stress situation and then be upset if they don't respond similarly. By understanding the effects of stress on performance, you have greater flexibility in dealing with intense situations.

This book is not about general stress, life stress, or career stress per se. However, it is important to realize that ongoing levels of stress in your life can affect acute stress responses. High levels of chronic stress can accelerate stress reactions in high-stress situations. Balance in your personal life is crucial.

Fear

Fear is a response related to sympathetic arousal. It is also a topic that is not discussed as much as it should be in nursing. Solomon (1990) defines fear as an automatic emotional reaction to a perceived danger or threat characterized by a high state of arousal. While there are some individuals who, in most situations, experience little or even no fear, these individuals are the exception. In fact, Rachman (1990) raises the interesting point that it may not be possible to demonstrate courage without feeling fear. He suggests that while these individuals may be fearless, this is not the same as courage, which requires feeling, confronting, and overcoming fear. Feeling no fear can carry its own problematic consequences.

Fear is our emotional equivalent of warning alarms. For our purposes, fear can be seen as the ultimate stress. It involves excessive arousal that can inhibit effective functioning. However, fear also has positive aspects. It can function to produce a readiness to respond, and, more importantly, it can signal the need for caution in certain situations.

Fear can show itself in different ways. Many of the symptoms of stress are the same as those of fear, though for the latter, they are often more intense, i.e., the hand tremor from stress becomes uncontrolled shaking from fear. There are also different types of fear.

This is important to recognize, as different types of fear have different approaches to mastery. The chart below lists

Psychological Techniques for Managing Fear

Realistic Fear	Fear of the Unknown	Anxiety	Illogical Fear	Fear of Failure	Fun Fear
Increased/Adjusted Training	Imaging Alternate Responses	PMR	Self-talk	Shaping	None Needed
Goal-Setting	Time to Explore	Tactical Breathing	Negative Thought Stopping	Self-Talk	
Imagery	Simulation	Biofeedback		VMBR	
Simulation				Counseling	

different types of fear and potential training and intervention approaches. Many of these, like progressive muscle relaxation (PMR) and visuo-motor-behavior-rehearsal (VMBR) are discussed in more detail later.

Realistic fears have a basis in reality, as there is a potential for pain, injury, or death if performance is inadequate. Realistic fears may be related to specific skills or situations. Each specific, realistic fear should suggest its own solution.

Realistic fears are often a sign that more training is needed. Remember, stress occurs when one doesn't feel prepared to meet the challenge of a given situation. These fears tend to subside with training and experience, which builds confidence. Other factors that can fuel realistic fears include past failure, negative or traumatic experiences, and improper or inadequate training experiences.

Increased training can help, but more of the same isn't always better. A different approach and/or different techniques may be needed. Simulation training is always an excellent tool, especially if integrated with mindset training, which might be called Mindset Infused Simulation Training (MIST).

Setting appropriate and achievable goals during training can help prevent or minimize fear. Performance-enhancing mental imagery (discussed later) can also be helpful in creating confidence for dealing with unlikely, unforeseen, or unusual, but worrisome situations.

Fear of the unknown is a specific form of realistic fear. Not knowing what to expect is frightening, though the anticipation of a situation is often worse than the actual situation itself. Experience is the best antidote for fear of the unknown. In fact, it's recognized that what makes an 'expert' isn't so much being smarter than anyone else, but rather having more experience in a given area. An expert knows what they are looking at, and because they have seen similar situations so many times before, they can quickly and effectively respond. The unknown has become well-known.

Fear of the unknown is also related to the uneasy or often terrifying 'What-If 'question.

What if:

- I screw up?

- Someone dies?
- I don't react quickly enough?
- I don't pick up on symptoms that are so obvious to everyone else?

'What-If' queries, especially if not answered, create anxiety and stress. When 'What-If' questions enter your mind, they should always be answered, even if the answer is not easy, preferred, or pleasant. Answering this type of question provides a plan and reduces the fear that would linger if the question remained unanswered. Always answer any what-if question with the best available plan and intervention.

For example, "what if you don't react quickly enough?" Sure, a situation may turn bad, or get worse, or emergent. BUT, that doesn't mean, it will be tragic (even though that is where your what-if thinking may take you). Further, as a nurse you have colleagues or other team members to back you up. We usually don't care for patients in a vacuum, so even if you don't perform your best, you usually have help.

This is why you need to recognize your 'what-if' thinking and prepare to answer its call. By the time you're an experienced nurse, hopefully, you're well enough prepared to react quickly in almost any situation. But even then, you may need a 'Plan B' to deal with the unexpected.

Simulation can be an extremely useful approach for fear of the unknown, as well. Sometimes just having time to explore or be in fearful situations at one's own pace can reduce uneasiness. Simply working with or having time to explore new equipment can begin to create greater comfort. Performance-enhancing mental imagery can also be useful in preparing for unknown or unusual situations by confronting them by mentally rehearsing responses to them.

Language can be important in managing what-if fears. Self-talk is discussed in depth later. However, as an example, it is useful to change the what-if proposition to an 'If-Then' statement: If X occurs, then I will… even better is a "when-then" statement: When X occurs, then I will. Such phraseology conveys greater certainty and specificity.

Anxiety isn't strictly a type of fear, but it is related to it. It is sometimes said that fear occurs when there is uneasiness about a specific object or situation, whereas anxiety is a diffuse uneasiness (fear) without a specific focus. Anxiety can also be seen as arousal that has become too intense or occurs from the wrong sources (unrelated to the immediate challenge).

There can also be a 'secondary anxiety.' This is anxiety about having anxiety. If you know and worry that becoming anxious can affect performance, this may actually create its own anxiety. This is often made worse when a nurse believes that they should never feel any anxiety or anxiety-related arousal, particularly in an emergency situation. Of course, this is unlikely, unreasonable, and unwise; and as we have discussed previously, some arousal is needed to perform well. However, if you (incorrectly) believe that there should be no uneasiness at all, the first signs of any degree of arousal can precipitate a rush of anxiety. The key is to understand arousal and anxiety and manage the arousal, not necessarily prevent or eliminate it.

Fear and anxiety can also result from being advanced too quickly in your career. A nurse may appear to have objectively good clinical skills, but may need more training or supervision before feeling comfortable in all situations and especially those that are emergent. This can be seen, for example, if you are pulled to cover a different floor with which you are not familiar. Or, if you are placed in a setting where you're 'it,' and you don't have all the backup you're accustomed to, you may feel an anxiety you've never felt before.

The nature of the anxiety should help suggest a solution. Stress management techniques like Progressive Muscle Relaxation, Performance-Enhancing Breathing, or Biofeedback can be useful for managing the symptoms of anxiety or a high level of sympathetic arousal. Adequate training, simulations, and recognizing anxiety and secondary anxiety can also prevent a negative impact on performance.

Illogical fear is fear that is out of proportion to objective realities and is often seen in self-doubts that are greater than what they should be. Illogical fears result from a distortion (usually an exaggeration) in perceptions of a situation. Nurses experiencing illogical fear use words like 'never' or 'always' when referring to a situation or themselves.

Comments such as "I always screw up when X is present" or "I never do well with Y procedure" represent illogical fear.

It's illogical because human beings rarely 'never' or 'always' do something, including screwing up. Words like 'never' and 'always' are excessive exaggerations, but are so powerful that they create fear and concern. The use of self-talk and negative thought-stopping can be helpful in managing illogical fears.

Fear of failure is a complicated fear, but it is not uncommon among highly motivated and achieving individuals. This is because high motivation can come from one of two sources: The Motive to Achieve Success (MAS) or The Motive to Avoid Failure (MAF), described by Atkinson (1964) and McClelland (1968). While both of these can produce high levels of commitment and effort, there are big differences in how they relate to performance and affect the individual.

If you are driven by the MAS (the motive to achieve success):

- You enjoy challenges.
- You don't mind problems and actually like to solve them.
- You don't mind setbacks because they just drive you harder.

- You enjoy the process of meeting challenges to see what you're capable of doing.
- You like seeing the outcome of your effort.
- You volunteer for new activities, and you're the first to try new things.

If you're driven by the MAF (the motive to avoid failure), you also work hard to succeed, but not because you enjoy the challenges and seek success. Instead:

- You're motivated because you fear and because you want to avoid the embarrassment of failing.
- You perform, but do so under great pressure, discomfort, and worry.
- Setbacks and changes are perceived as horrific catastrophes because they impede your reaching your goal, and they raise the specter of failure.
- You don't enjoy the process of overcoming the challenge.
- You strive for the relief of obtaining a successful outcome and being done.

> You tend not to volunteer for new activities as this only puts more pressure on you.

> You don't enjoy your accomplishments as much as you feel relief that you made it through without screwing up too badly.

Most nurses, like most people, are a blend of both MAS and MAF. Much of this is related to our experiences while growing up and experiences during training. Positive training, the kind that emphasizes development, tends to foster MAS, while negative, critical, or failure-based training fosters MAF.

Dealing with the fear of failure can be quite complicated because its roots penetrate deeply into one's development. At a minimum, it requires understanding that mistakes are part of learning and they present an opportunity for improvement. It also requires separating one's self-concept and self-worth from a single performance situation. "Never judge yourself by your worst day" (Grossman, 2004).

A specific technique to try is 'shaping' skills, i.e., learning skills in small achievable steps to experience success. A positive training philosophy can also be effective in mediating fear of failure, and aspects of cognitive therapy such as addressing self-talk and performance-degrading thoughts, can help at times, as well. Other times, more formal psychotherapy is needed.

Fun fear is found in thrill activities like riding rollercoasters and skydiving. Actually, so-called "fun fear" more accurately represents an activity that induces arousal rather than fear. Certainly, arousal can be pleasurable, and indeed, many individuals choose to work in the ED or as paramedics because they enjoy the feelings of arousal. Emergency responders, especially pre-hospital providers, often label themselves 'adrenaline junkies.'

However, there is a difference between fun fear/arousal and actual fear. Fun fear has the common element of control and mastery. Fun fear assumes the rollercoaster, despite its speed, will not jump its tracks. It assumes that despite the danger when jumping from an airplane, the parachute or, at least, the secondary parachute will open. Actual fear only occurs when these things are out of control.

Despite the frequency of fear and the existence of techniques for its management, it's well-recognized that controlling fear isn't always easy to do. The primary barrier to mastering fear is denial of fear's existence, something that nurses often do for many reasons, not the least of which is embarrassment. Your fear may come from the (erroneous) belief that no other nurse has experienced such feelings. You may be worried about looking weak, not having the 'right stuff,' or being seen as incompetent by others.

The second barrier to mastering fear is the denial or denigration of fear by others, especially faculty, colleagues, or supervisors. Even more unfortunate, despite being in a position to teach or help nurses understand and manage fear, they neglect to do so. This avoidance may stem from the same reasons that make an individual reluctant to discuss fear. It may result from a faulty understanding of human psychological function or the lack of understanding of how to deal with the fear issue. Whether from macho philosophy, embarrassment, or ignorance as to what to offer others to help manage fear (other than comments like 'get over it'), the issue is too often ignored.

Professionals who work with addictions often talk about the problem in the family being like an "elephant in the living room." There is this gigantic disruption in their lives that they try to ignore, avoid and deny, but the addiction clearly impacts everyone. Fear in emergency situations is much like that elephant. The key is to acknowledge, understand, manage, and use the natural emotion of fear. Famous test pilot Chuck Yeager is quoted as saying:

> *I was always afraid of dying. Always. It was my fear that made me learn everything I could about my airplane and my emergency equipment and kept me flying, respectful of my machine, and always alert in the cockpit.*

A friend and fire chief respected for his performance excellence captured a philosophy of accepting and transforming fear by saying:

> *You replace fear of a situation with respect for its challenges.*

If you respect the challenges of a situation, you will prepare for it, and when prepared, performance stress will be less likely.

Managing Arousal, Stress, and Fear: A Preview

Given that reactions in high-stress situations can be normal but problematic for nurses, it is essential to control and minimize them. As noted, experience is the usual way adaptation to stress occurs. Individuals who are experienced with a given set of skills show a different pattern of arousal from those who are less experienced with the same set.

This classic figure from research by Fenz and Epstein (1967) shows the pattern of arousal between experienced skydivers and inexperienced skydivers.

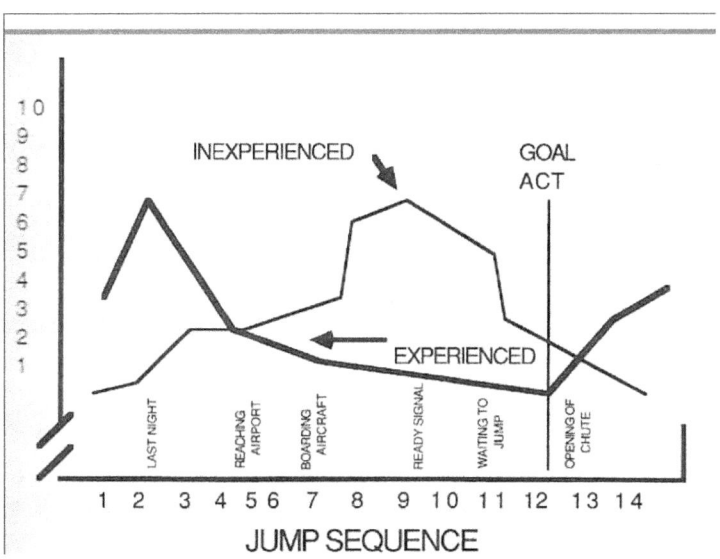

Note that inexperienced skydivers have rather low levels of arousal when there is still considerable time until the jump (the night before). But as they prepare, approach the airport, begin their ascent in the plane, and receive the ready signal, their level of arousal increases significantly. After the jump is (safely) over, arousal declines once more…in a sense of relief.

For experienced skydivers, however, the pattern is different. Their arousal is actually higher the night before as they enthusiastically anticipate the jump. As they approach the airport, board the plane, ascend, and receive the ready signal, they gain control over their arousal as they focus on their mental checklist, just as a pilot goes over the preflight checklist. The experienced skydivers' levels of arousal decrease with this focus until after the chute opens, and they then feel the exhilaration of the jump. This is a typical pattern found in many areas of human performance when comparing experienced performers with novices. Inexperienced individuals become m more anxious as a critical point nears; experienced individuals focus on the task and manage their arousal.

Of course, becoming experienced requires time and assumes an adequate number of general emergency experiences and emergencies of the same type for familiarization with their nature. Additionally, the emergency response must have gone well, or at least, not been traumatic. Unfortunately, despite many similarities in emergencies, there are so many possible differences that it can take quite a while to become an expert in even one kind.

Simulation or reality-based scenario training and performance-enhancing mental imagery are excellent approaches to gaining experience and exposure to various types of emergency situations. Repeated training can help dampen arousal and strengthen emotional control. Unfortunately, time and access may limit training of this nature. Therefore, using the psychological skills described next chapters add another dimension to your nursing training for performance excellence by developing a greater level of control and self-regulation of emotion and arousal.

V. Mental Valium: Sympathetic Modulation and Performance

Keep calm and Nightingale on.

- Scrubsmag.com

The goal of The Code Calm Mindset psychological skills training is to maximize performance under stress. The challenge in a medical emergency is control; control of the clinical situation, control of the emergency response, and control of yourself. This is accomplished in two different, but related ways. One is by controlling sympathetic arousal and its performance-degrading effects. It, therefore, indirectly enhances performance. The second approach applies psychological techniques to directly optimize performance skills.

We'll begin by discussing sympathetic arousal, of which there are two types. Under-arousal and over-arousal.

Insufficient Sympathetic Arousal

Given the nature of the stress response, self-regulation techniques are needed and typically have the goal of reducing the excessive sympathetic arousal that is often innate to such situations. Using these techniques gives you the sympathetic modulation skills to down-regulate. However, there are times when under-arousal, or too little arousal, is the problem.

These are times when you need to increase your sympathetic arousal or *up-regulate*. This might occur when you are tired at the end of a busy shift, bored on an extended shift, or when it's just 'one of those days' when you're just 'not into it.'

Being tired at the end of a busy shift can cause arousal to drop below levels where performance is optimal. You may have been on your game earlier in the shift, but the combination of patients was particularly challenging, so now you're at the end of your rope. That morning coffee and afternoon Monster drink only went so far, and now your thoughts are on giving reports, wrapping up paperwork, and going home.

Boredom can occur anytime, depending on the nature of your patient load. Call bell after call bell can lull you into a sense of complacency. Pick your least favorite minor patient complaint, and after you've seen a few on a given shift, the last thing you're expecting is runs of ventricular tachycardia in a seemingly stable patient. Worse still, is being both bored and fatigued on the same shift.

We all have natural variations in alertness, mood, and enthusiasm for work. There are days when you just start feeling like your performance is less than ideal. If emergency action is required on one of those days when you're just not into it, adequate arousal may be absent. An 'off day' may be inconsequential in some jobs, but it can lead to serious consequences in nursing care. Maybe distractions at home are contributing to your lack of zeal for work. Maybe preparing for a clinical presentation or studying for a licensing exam is weighing on your mind. Whatever the case may be, techniques to boost arousal may be useful.

Another common situation where maintaining sympathetic arousal (if not increasing it) can be crucial is when a critical situation case seems to be stabilized. This can be a time of great surprise, stress, and sub-optimal performance if your focus and readiness are relaxed too soon. You stabilized the patient and called the ICU when suddenly, your patient crashes again. Reversing gears is not easy and especially since you're working against natural physiological responses. This was cautioned by Napoleon, who said:

The moment of greatest vulnerability is the instant after victory.

Combine this with the observation of Doss (1994), who notes the effects after an intense response are both physical and psychological:

Exhaustion and confusion are typical after-effects from being involved in a high-stress situation, even for trained individuals.

Feeling that the worst is over and that disaster has been avoided has been called the 'Whew Factor' by Gonzalez (2003). Wiping your brow and letting out a 'Whew' sigh of relief is common. But, he cautions that this letting down of one's guard may occur prematurely. So, to quote the famous New York Yankee Yogi Berra again:

It ain't over 'til it's over.

All of these situations call for you to have means to increase your physiological arousal, and there are a variety of ways to do that. They include:

- Physical warm-ups
- Cue words
- Cue images
- Attentional focus
- Rituals
- Self-efficacy statements
- Anger transformation
- Music
- Physical Presence/ Embodied Cognition

While not purely a psychological technique, physical warm-ups can be useful for increasing arousal. Remembering that the mind and body are connected, physical activation can spur psychological activation, as well. This doesn't mean you should do jumping jacks in the nurses' station or wind sprints down the hall. This can be as simple as air squats, neck rotations, arm circles, and the like. Even a small amount of physical exercise to stretch and raise your heart rate a little can help raise your arousal level. The start of a shift (and at various points during a shift) can provide opportunities for brief warm-ups.

Cue words are words or phrases you say to yourself to increase energy. Examples might be: 'focus,' 'react,' 'think,' 'clear,' 'plan,' or 'ABCs.' Being taught as the classic algorithm for ACLS and ATLS, saying *'airway, breathing, circulation'* to yourself can also put you in the right frame of mind to act accordingly. They are likely already etched in your mind, so remembering them is not difficult.

Usually, cue words are said quietly or internally to yourself. However, a study by Hunziker et al. (2013) suggested that external expression may help focus and respond in a crisis. They found that expressing two questions out loud during simulated cardiopulmonary resuscitation, "What is the patient's condition?" and "What immediate action is needed?" decreased perceived stress without negatively affecting performance.

Cue images are mind pictures and mind movies of you responding well. We will discuss this in much more depth as part of performance-enhancing mental imagery. But for now, know that mental rehearsal is a powerful preparation and performance enhancement technique. Cue images may also be images of your body being ready to respond. Feeling confidence "flow" in your hands or seeing your brain "light up and electrically charge" may seem silly at first, but it has been used successfully to induce readiness to respond.

Attentional focus means to consciously focus on the emergency skills at hand. It's a conscious attempt to block out irrelevant thoughts and bring all your energy to bear on your response. Attentional focus is often facilitated by the use of an actual or mental *'checklist'* of what needs to be done in a given situation. The simplest form of this is seen in students who make sure they have all their books and materials before going to class. Similarly, pilots go over a checklist before every flight.

And this same type of communication has been used to avoid errors in the operating room.

Most athletes go through certain rituals to 'psych up' and prepare themselves for competition. It's essential for you to do the same, but in preparation for your response to potential emergency situations rather than competition. You can do this by mentally preparing for each shift in general. At some point, you need to make the transformation from an 'at-home' mindset to a 'focused-ready' mindset when you start your patient responsibilities. You want to be able to 'throw a switch' that increases your readiness. It's your choice whether it happens when you walk out of your house, enter the hospital, arrive on your floor, don your scrubs, or any other point you choose – as long as you prepare yourself at some appropriate time.

Self-efficacy statements like: "I'm feeling ready" and "I'm feeling sharp" are used to instill a powerful sense of confidence. You may feel awkward at first saying these things to yourself, but they can have a strong impact on your readiness. This can certainly help counter negative self-talk that we will discuss later.

Anger transformation is used by some individuals to help energize themselves by getting angry or 'ticked off' about something and then drawing on this energy to respond. Providers might induce arousal by getting angry at the illness or injury or being determined to not 'get beat' by the injuries or not lose the patient. However, there is certainly some controversy about using anger as a self-regulation technique for psyching up, so we'll touch on it here only briefly.

It was the great baseball player, Pittsburgh Pirate, Roberto Clemente, who said:

If I would be happy, I would be a very bad ballplayer. With me, when I get mad, it puts energy in my body.

The problem is that the amount of anger/energy produced can be unpredictable and uncontrollable. Additionally, being angry during a response can be distracting or disruptive. In a team environment like the ED, OR, or ICU, that can be a big problem. The iconic New York Yankee Lou Gehrig recognized the deleterious effect of anger:

... the ball player who "loses his head and can't keep his cool" is worse than no player at all.

Goleman (1997) provides further support that anger may not be the best psychological preparation technique. He says that catharsis (getting anger out) may be a problem because, contrary to what many believe, it does not dispel anger. It actually pumps up the brain and prolongs thinking about the anger situation. Your anger may trigger or set off an aggressive response towards you in colleagues that might not have otherwise occurred and may result in interpersonal friction and even impaired team performance.

Cultivating anger as motivation or preparation can become a habit that makes you unable to generally 'play well with others' in any setting, even at home. And the impact on home and other personal and professional situations may be considerable, as the anger may be difficult to mute, let alone dispel, after you have been cultivating it for an entire shift. Finally, anger as a chronic style may not only cause you interpersonal issues, but health problems as well.

If anger works well for you, okay. Just know that this is a controversial self-management approach that is generally not recommended. Research (Murphy, 2005) suggests anger may increase performance on strength-related tasks for some individuals (those who have strong physiological responses to anger imagery). However, the data are not conclusive, and brute strength is generally not a requirement for precise nursing emergency skills.

Music is the most popular method of psyching up among athletes: hard-pounding rhythms to get up and mellow tunes to relax. Nursing emergencies rarely allow time to use music, but it might be useful to prepare before your shift or during a quick break on a busy night. Alternatively, you can use music to relax or get to sleep in order to prepare for the next day. It is not necessary to have the music coming through your $300 BOSE or BEATS headphones; simply thinking about (or singing to yourself) a song that elevates your mood has an effect. In fact, it may be good to select, develop and practice your 'pump it up' song so you have it when you need it.

Another useful technique is physical presence. Physical presence is how you physically present yourself in a challenging situation. It is very powerful in influencing behavior. One impact of what is commonly termed non-verbal behavior is its significant effect on others' perceptions of your mood, confidence, and potential actions. An aspect of this called *embodied cognition* proposes that your posture and presentation also affect your own mood, confidence, and actions.

Dr. Amy Cuddy at Harvard University is an expert in the physical expressions of behavior and, specifically, impressions of dominance. Her research finds that just like in the animal world, human dominance is represented by certain posturing (the peacock spreading tailfeathers, the cat hissing, etc.). She has found that when human beings 'power pose' by standing straight up, making themselves 'big' and expanding their presence, a message of confidence is conveyed to others, but as importantly, also to yourself. The opposite can also be true that looking downward, drooping your shoulders, and scrunching up sends messages of submission and incompetence.

The effect is both psychological and physiological, as she found that power posing increases an individual's level of testosterone (which she calls the dominance hormone) and decreases the level of cortisol (which she labels the stress hormone). Therefore, she suggests that power posing (in private!) prior to entering a stressful, critical, or evaluative situation can positively affect a person's confidence (Cuddy, 2015; Cuddy, 2016).

Power posing needs to be used judiciously. Obviously, engaging in the akimbo pose (the 'superman' or superwoman-like stance of hands on hips, chest out, and head and eyes raised to the sky) may be useful for mental preparation, but wholly inappropriate displayed on the floor or in a patient's room. There is controversy over these findings, but the message here is that how you present yourself, especially in a frightened or unsure posture, can influence not only others' perception of you, but also your perception of yourself and how you will respond.

Once you've mastered some of these techniques, it's useful to share them with those around you. You don't work in a vacuum. Virtually every crisis situation in the hospital or emergency department will have a team of people responding to it. It will often be your job to lead, and you can use some of these techniques to focus everyone's attention on the task at hand and maximize their response and the outcome.

Excessive Sympathetic Arousal

Because of the stress inherent in emergency events, the more common problem is excessive sympathetic arousal, getting too 'hyped up' or energized. The sympathetic modulation goal here is to *down-regulate*.

Effective techniques for down-regulation include:

- The Relaxation Response
- Meditation
- Yoga
- Imagery
- Self-Hypnosis
- Autogenic Training
- Biofeedback
- Progressive Muscle Relaxation
- Relaxation Imagery
- Performance-Enhancing Breathing Techniques
- Visuo-Motor Behavioral Rehearsal
- Stress Inoculation Training

We will describe these approaches only briefly here, as many require specific education and training. Further, many of these techniques require this training, practice, and familiarity BEFORE they are applied in high-intensity crisis situations. However, it is valuable to be aware of these techniques, and if you take time to gain ability with them, they can be invaluable in helping you perform optimally when you need to be at your best.

These techniques and other concepts and approaches discussed in this book can be pursued through discussion with psychologists, psychiatrists, or others likely to be on your hospital staff. However, whichever professional you choose, be sure to ascertain that they truly understand the techniques and their application to performance enhancement and not just clinical problems.

The Relaxation Response

The Relaxation Response is a form of 'Americanized' meditation developed by Dr. Herbert Benson (1975) of the Mind-Body Institute and Harvard Medical School. The relaxation response involves sitting comfortably in a quiet setting and repeating a word or phrase that suggests relaxation to you. In traditional meditation, this word or phrase called your mantra, is usually spoken in Hindu, though any word or phrase suggesting calmness, relaxation, and focus can be used.

This is a passive method of inducing relaxation, meaning that it's important to focus on the word or phrase and let the relaxation happen. You cannot force it, which many people try to do. Relaxation involves "letting go" to allow a calmer state to evolve. Forcing is the opposite of this.

Initially, the relaxation response was created to help treat people with refractory hypertension. Because of its success in this area, it has been applied to other stress-related disorders, such as tension headaches and those situations where a state of relaxation is desired to help treat or cope with the problem situation. Dr. Benson has done some fascinating and important research on the power of meditative techniques, which is discussed in more detail shortly.

Mindfulness and Meditation

Meditation and the contemporary term of mindfulness evolved from ancient Eastern techniques that are highly effective ways to control and quiet the body. In fact, it was the practitioners of these arts who taught Western medicine that it's possible for an individual to control functions in the body that were thought to be only controllable by medication, such as heart rate, blood pressure, and muscle tightness. These were named 'autonomic responses,' as it was believed they were automatic and could not be controlled by the individual.

Interestingly, Begley (2007) feels that the musical group The Beatles helped legitimize the scientific study of meditation and yoga in Western medicine. In 1968, the four Beatles went to study with the Maharishi Yogi, a journey well covered by the press. Begley writes, "Their visit popularized the notion that the spiritual East has something to teach the rational West."

Meditation is based on concentrating or chanting a mantra. While still controversial, some research suggests that several forms of meditation can improve concentration, reaction time, learning, and memory (Walsh & Shapiro, 2006).

Dr. Herbert Benson and his Harvard team, in developing the relaxation response discussed above, studied the ability of Tibetan monks to use a form of meditation called Tum-Mo to master metabolic and other physiological bodily processes

(Cromie, 2002). Demonstrations of uncanny ability took place in northern India in a chilly room of forty degrees Fahrenheit.

After the monks entered a state of deep meditation, they were draped in wet sheets that had been soaked in cold water (49 degrees F). Rather than developing the hypothermia and uncontrolled shivering that would affect most of us, the monks continued to meditate with little reaction. More remarkably, steam began to rise from them as the cold sheets reacted to the meditating monks' body heat.

In other studies, the monks warmed the temperature of their toes and fingers by as much as seventeen degrees. They were also able to slow their metabolism through meditation by sixty-four percent. For comparison, when we sleep, our metabolism slows about ten to fifteen percent. Other forms of simple meditation find metabolic decreases of about seventeen percent.

The current frequently used term and popular form of meditation is mindfulness or mindfulness-based stress reduction. Developed and popularized by Dr. Jonathan Kabat-Zinn, it is described as "Awareness that arises through paying attention, on purpose, in the present moment, non-judgmentally" (Kabat-Zinn, 2016). Much like traditional meditation, it creates a focus on the here and now to block stress-inducing distractions.

Yoga

Yoga is based on rhythmic breathing techniques in conjunction with dynamic body postures. Yoga practices have been beneficial in training concentration and conditioning the body to avoid or even treat muscle injury from uncomfortable or contorted positions that can occur in emergency circumstances and in providing care to patients.

While yoga, meditation, and mindfulness are widely accepted today, those who remain skeptical should be aware that ancient warriors used techniques like yoga to prepare for combat by developing physical prowess and mental discipline. Modern warriors train in these techniques to maximize their performance under stress.

Self-Hypnosis

The word hypnosis should no longer bring up images of a stage hypnotist making subjects cluck like chickens or act in an embarrassing manner or images of an exotic swami putting people under a spell. There certainly has been an ever-greater acceptance of the value of hypnosis in clinical medicine (Elkins, 2016).

Self-hypnosis is not magic, but a form of concentration control. In hypnosis, one area of focus is so strong that everything else seems blocked out. Nowicki (1994) defines it as a 'state of relaxation characterized by heightened awareness, restricted mental focus, and increased suggestibility.'

We often engage in a form of self-hypnosis in our daily lives through distraction. For example, if we ask you how your shoes feel, you could tell us if they are comfortable, tight, or pinching. Chances are that prior to our asking, you were not thinking about them at all; you didn't even feel your shoes or your feet. But, of course, they were there, and had you needed to jump up and act, you could have done so without a problem. The distraction of your attention away from your feet (by reading and concentrating on this book…or by daydreaming) is a form of self-hypnosis. It is the act of concentrating so intently that other distractions are blocked-out.

Another example of a hypnotic-like state you may have experienced is being bored on a long car trip. It often occurs that rather than tedious, boring miles crawling by, all of a sudden you realize multiple miles and many minutes have gone by in what felt like no time at all. Distraction "shrunk" the tedious time for you. The key is to develop self-hypnosis as a skill through practice rather than have it occur by happenstance.

Autogenic Training

Autogenic training is a technique developed in Germany in the early part of the last century that uses self-suggestions of warmth and heaviness in your body to induce relaxation (Schultz & Luthe, 1959). You begin in a quiet setting and relaxed position and make self-suggestions of body regulation. For example, you would say: "My arms and legs are heavy and warm." "My heart rate is slow, calm, and regular." These are repeated several times, consciously feeling the heaviness and feeling the calmness. You can also use calming statements, such as 'I am at peace' (Lichtenstein, 1988).

Biofeedback

Biofeedback is another self-regulation technique that has seen increasing acceptance and use in treating clinical conditions, especially stress-related illnesses (Schwartz & Andrasik, 2017). Biofeedback incorporates any relaxation technique but informs you via a biofeedback instrument (machine) if your body is actually responding and relaxing.

In biofeedback, a device attached to your body measures a physiological response related to stressed or relaxed states. Typical forms of biofeedback include heart rate and blood pressure monitors, galvanic skin response, muscle tightness, skin temperature, and EEG alpha wave tracking. Biofeedback systems can monitor a single body reaction or several body responses at the same time.

Consider this question: When you get stressed, does your skin temperature go up or down (warm or cool)?

The answer is that stress decreases skin temperature in your hands and, hence, creates the 'cold sweat' you feel in your palms. Warmer skin temperature is associated with relaxation and reduced stress.

In biofeedback, while you practice a relaxation technique, the biofeedback device gives you information as to whether your body is responding and, if so, how much. For example, you learn to raise your skin temperature using a relaxation technique enhanced by cues (lights or sounds corresponding to increased or decreased skin temperature) from the instrument. Since it's impossible to be stressed and relaxed simultaneously, learning to control and raise your skin temperature can help prevent or abort a stress response.

Biofeedback is widely used in training athletes. Biofeedback is used to make athletes more aware of and in control of specific physiological reactions in their bodies during performance (Helin & Sihvonen, 1987; Janelle, Hillman, et al., 2000). Biofeedback has been used to help astronauts learn self-regulation for managing the stress of extended missions and to maintain attention (Pope & Prinzel, n.d.).

Progressive Muscle Relaxation

Unlike some forms of relaxation training that are largely cognitive and passive, Progressive Muscle Relaxation (PMR) is a physically and mentally active approach. This fits better with the more action-oriented nature of many nurses, especially those most likely to be involved in emergency care. It provides a good point of focus and is shown to be superior to other relaxation techniques.

Traditional PMR has its roots in the work of Dr. Edmund Jacobson in the 1920's and is a simple technique. It begins with tensing and then relaxing different muscle groups in the body. For example, you start by tensing and then relaxing muscles in your hands and arms, then your shoulders and neck, followed by your chest and stomach, and finally your legs, feet, and toes. The initial training session takes about fifteen to twenty minutes. Once mastered, you move to the next level, called 'letting go.' This involves relaxing without tensing the muscles first; you just let go of the tension.

PMR works because tensing and relaxing the muscles trains them to relax and release tension. When muscles relax, other parts of the body respond, as well. Heart rate slows, blood pressure decreases, and breathing becomes slower and easier. Training in PMR also helps you recognize signs of tension in your muscles, whether from stress, posture, or both. Initiating relaxation at the earliest signs of muscle tension makes it easier to reverse it, rather than waiting until tension is high and muscles are already extremely tense.

The process of psychological conditioning allows PMR, once well-trained, to work fast, sometimes in a matter of seconds. This involves associating muscle relaxation with a cue word or phrase that you say or think to yourself. (This may also be referred to as a 'key' or 'trigger.') This can be any word or phrase as long as it suggests relaxation and calmness.

Words like 'focus,' 'smooth,' 'easy,' or 'relax' can be used. In traditional and clinical PMR, using words like 'Hawaii' or 'Blue Sky' helps create relaxation. However, it is probably best that nurses not think about white sands and fluffy clouds in the middle of a code. So, choose a cue word that fits better with the environment and the action of emergency care like those suggested above.

Focusing on the cue word while creating relaxation in your body and mind creates an association (a conditioned response) between that cue word and controlled relaxation in your body. With practice, just thinking the cue word or whispering it will cue the start of your relaxation. You will not have to spend fifteen minutes tensing/relaxing muscles to achieve relaxation. Thinking or uttering your cue word will be like flipping on a light switch or a relaxation switch to create a more relaxed state.

An alternate term for the cue or keyword is of 'anchor.' Anchors are cues that recall patterns of behavior (Alexander, et al., 1990). It is useful to realize that anchors can be verbal, visual, or physical. For example, relaxation cueing can be enhanced by associating a physical anchor with the relaxation training or the keyword. Making a fist, extending the fingers, or touching a particular spot on the body would be examples of physical anchors that could be conditioned and used to recall and stimulate relaxed states. An image can also be an anchor.

There are some cautions that should be mentioned in regard to relaxation training. First, mastering relaxation and creating effective conditioning takes practice both to develop and maintain. Secondly, relaxation is a fundamental skill; it is not a cure-all or substitute for other skill training. You have to be smart about the application of this training, especially if you become very good at producing relaxation. Use caution so that you don't produce excessive relaxation before or during an emergency situation. While it's unlikely that this would happen, remember your goal is to be in your O-ZONE. Use relaxation as part of the process to achieve it.

Relaxation techniques are usually without side effects, and although they are used to treat many medical and psychological conditions, if you have a health concern, it is best to check with your own physician before intensely pursuing relaxation training. This is especially true if you have a history of trauma-related psychological problems or post-traumatic stress disorder.

There are many benefits to developing self-regulation via PMR. They include the ability to:

- Control the physiology of stress
- Reduce anxiety about critical performance
- Reduce stress impacts on thinking
- Enhance other skills and learning
- Conserve energy while waiting to start intervening
- Regain energy during or after an emergency
- Manage anger or frustration
- Promote sleep

Your objective here is to get control over the physiology of stress. Where you feel stress, PMR helps to manage and reduce it. Being relaxed facilitates thinking and concentration and prevents brain-lock. Although we are focusing on the application of PMR related to medical emergencies, the regular practice of relaxation enhances general stress resistance in other areas of your life. Finally, a relaxed state can help in all types of learning, as this enhances attention to and retention of material and skills.

While many emergencies require instantaneous intervention, it is not unusual that a medical emergency response may take some time to set up or stage, as in a trauma alert. Because of the conditioned arousal of the alert and the motivation 'to get at it,' arousal can quickly peak and be very high, though there is a delay in initiation. This 'being stuck in neutral' with 'your engine revving' can lead to a quick drain of energy before a lengthy resuscitation process even begins.

A more relaxed state helps prevent anger and frustration. If these destructive emotions are already present, relaxation can help reduce their intensity. Maybe other staff are not responding as quickly as you expect; maybe other team members disagree with your approach; maybe an attending has just criticized what you are doing. You feel like exploding as your frustration increases.

PMR can help you manage that frustration and even anger more effectively so that you focus or assert yourself without overreacting in a way that gets you written off, escorted from the OR, or worse. Whether your anger or frustration is because of that particular situation, with yourself, or for some other reason, relaxation can reduce those feelings and help you refocus on the needs of the moment.

During those lengthy shifts and extremely busy days, you may want a break or need to recharge; use relaxation for personal rehab and recuperation. Remember the importance of R&R, reset, and recovery periods. Nowicki (1997) reports that Russian sports psychologists have for some time endorsed relaxation techniques as a way to speed the recovery of ability during breaks in the competition. Relaxation promotes deeper breathing, greater muscle relaxation, decreased fatigue, and decreased pain or discomfort.

While there is often a physical and physiological 'crash' after completing treatment on an emergent patient as a result of all the physical and mental energy expended, you might experience the opposite and feel charged with energy, especially after a successful high-stress response. This may make it difficult to return to more mundane tasks on the rest of your shift or get to sleep after your shift is over. Down-regulation and relaxation techniques help promote sleep more quickly in such situations so you can get the rest you need before duty calls again.

Relaxation has been associated with what has been called "the Eureka Effect," or having sudden insight into solving a problem. Do you ever have those moments right before you fall asleep when innovative ideas or solutions to problems flash in your mind? It's those moments of relaxation that allow the mind to find novel approaches to challenges.

The yelling of Eureka (which means 'I found it') upon finding a solution to a problem, having great insight, or discovering a desired object (as gold in California) can be traced back to the ancient Greek mathematician Archimedes (Alexander et al., 1990).

After much intense concentration and thought as to how to solve a challenge given to him by his king (i.e. how to determine how much actual gold was in the king's crown without melting it down), he was relaxing in his bath. He suddenly realized that gold would displace more water than other metals and jumped from the tub and ran naked down the city streets, yelling, "Eureka." This was an early example of how relaxation after intense concentration can promote insight and problem-solving.

Relaxation Imagery

Imagery has many applications in human performance. We already discussed imagery for increasing arousal when needed, and we will talk about skill-related performance-enhancing imagery in a later chapter. Imagery can also be used to down-regulate stress responses.

To put it simply, relaxation imagery is imagining a pleasant or relaxing scene. This approach is often joked about as 'going to your happy place.' However, calming, pleasant, and enjoyable images such as the beach or a lake or spending time with your family can induce such feelings in us by providing relaxing stimuli and by blocking out negative or stressful images.

Performance-Enhancing Breathing Techniques (PEBTs)

Performance–Enhancing Breathing Techniques comprise another set of effective techniques for managing medical emergency stress. There are many names for self-control breathing techniques and many forms. The point is that PEBTs are often quite useful in managing the arousal or stress of an emergency. Slow rhythmic breathing shifts the body into a more relaxed state.

Because breathing techniques can be so effective in managing stress and enhancing performance, Siddle (1995) suggested:

We would argue that breath control should be a mandatory component of survival stress management.

Diaphragmatic breathing is a particularly effective technique for arousal control. This method is called 'diaphragmatic' because it involves breathing anchored at your diaphragm. It has also been called 'belly breathing.' Breathing techniques are effective because they counteract the effects of disrupted breathing that occurs under stress.

Try the following: Count to three and then take a breath as quickly as you can. Hold it for about two seconds, exhale, and then return to breathing normally.

What did you notice? You might have been aware of several things. First, your breath (if inhaled quickly) probably was not very deep. Further, if you remember your posture, you probably felt your chest and shoulders tense and lift towards your ears until you exhaled.

What emotional state does this posture resemble? Most say it feels and looks like the state of being scared, surprised, or shocked. This muscle posturing that occurs with change from diaphragmatic to chest breathing is known as dysponesis and negatively affects breathing and comfort (Behavioral Physiology Institute, 2008).

Studies of dysfunctional breathing patterns find several things:

➤ There is a failure to breathe diaphragmatically.
➤ There is a failure to exhale completely.

➢ There is a failure to allow transition time between breaths.

➢ There is a failure to monitor breathing.

➢ There is the use of accessory muscles for breathing when not needed.

Diaphragmatic breathing has advantages over chest breathing. Chest breathing is described as inefficient, labor-intensive, and makes breathing seem difficult and even exhausting. In fact, most singers use diaphragmatic breathing to enhance projection and endurance when performing. Chest breathing negatively affects breathing efficiency in several ways:

➢ It requires breathing faster, leading to a sense of urgency or anxiety.

➢ It makes complete exhalation difficult, leading to a sense of tightness.

➢ It can lead to feelings of being confined or trapped.

➢ It can create a sense of struggle with breathing rather than relaxation.

It is cautioned that 'deep breathing' is not the be-all and end-all approach to managing stress. The key is slow, quiet, individualized breathing. Here is a way to develop or improve your diaphragmatic breathing skills:

- ➢ Place one hand palm down on your stomach and the other hand palm down on your chest. If you're chest breathing (the less effective type), you will see the hand on your chest rise and fall.
- ➢ Now, breathe deeply and low from your diaphragm. Notice your stomach distend and the hand on your stomach rise and fall.
- ➢ Or purse your lips together like you're breathing through a straw. This helps produce diaphragmatic breathing, as well.
- ➢ Or take quick sniffs of air to engage diaphragmatic breathing.

Diaphragmatic breathing tends to occur naturally when lying down on your back. From that position, look to see whether your stomach does indeed rise and fall more than your chest, an indication of diaphragmatic breathing.

Another effective technique is four-count breathing (also termed tactical, combat, or box breathing). It involves a slow inhale to the count of four, breath holds to the count of four, slow exhale to the count of four, and rest to the count of four prior to the next inhalation.

While these may be the most recognized techniques, there are multiple iterations such that sub-optimal success with one technique should not dissuade you from trying other approaches. The benefits of finding a breathing technique that works for you are physical, psychological, and performance-enhancing in many different ways (Vranich, 2016).

Whichever technique you decide on, you can use it in several ways. Let's use diaphragmatic breathing as an example. Whenever you start to notice that you're becoming stressed, take one or two diaphragmatic breaths to help *break the cycle* of increasing stress. You do not need to do diaphragmatic breathing all the time; only one or two breaths should work.

You can also develop a habit of taking one or two diaphragmatic breaths at various intervals during an emergency situation or a duty shift as a way to *prevent the build-up* of stress. This can also help remind you to monitor your stress levels as well as provide an 'automatic reset' of any stress you might be experiencing. Breathwork is an excellent foundation for implementing the R&R we discussed earlier. Breathing patterns where your exhale is longer than your inhale is the key to helping create calmness (Bertram, 2023).

PEBTs are useful not only because of their effectiveness, but also because they are easy to do and can be done 'covertly' in many different situations. In other words, you can control and relax yourself without anyone else being aware.

Centering

Centering is another breathing-related technique used to manage the stress of high-risk situations. It is well described by performance expert Dr. Robert Nideffer (Nideffer & Sharpe, 1978; Nideffer, 1985), who learned it while studying the martial art of Aikido in Japan. The purpose of centering is to develop a controlled state of relaxed focus, which, to use the Japanese simile, is a 'mind like still water.'

Centering begins by taking a diaphragmatic breath, but adds a centering image. You let all of your attention and focus come to rest at your 'center of gravity,' which is located about two inches behind your belly button. This means that as you let your eyes close, let all your awareness focus on this point. Sometimes this is experienced as looking out from behind your belly button. Open your eyes and return to your regular breathing and activity.

If this is a little too mystical for you, try a more Western approach. Let your eyes close and inhale slowly and deeply as in a diaphragmatic breath. Exhale and gently imagine a leaf or feather floating slowly, slowly drifting down…lower and lower…until it gently comes to rest, floating softly at your center of gravity (belly button). Open your eyes and return to your regular breathing and activity.

Initially, you should do this in a safe and quiet environment. However, like PMR, you will eventually develop the skill to do it quickly with your eyes open, in any position, focused but aware, even when all about you is chaotic. Adding a refocusing command, as described in the next section, 'Attention Control Training,' will further increase the effect of centering on your performance.

Attention Control Training (ACT)

Dr. Nideffer has also extended centering (Nideffer & Sharpe, 1978) into a technique called Attention Control Training (ACT). ACT is comprised of first completing the centering process: inhale and exhale with your centering image.

Then you give yourself a cue- a clinically relevant instruction or an intervention-relevant self-command- to refocus on what you need to do. For example, after centering, you might instruct yourself or issue a relevant self-command to "assess the airway" or "review the rhythm."

You can use ACT to regain focus:

➢ Should an unexpected event occur that distracts you

➢ When your stress increases to an uncomfortable level

➢ When you have made a mistake and your inability to 'shake it off' prevents you from further reacting to the immediate challenge in front of you

Sympathetic modulation, whether up-regulation or down-regulation, is a fundamental, but essential and powerful psychological performance skill well-worth mastering.

VI. Mental Scopes: Concentration Skills and Performance

For it may safely be said, not that the habit of ready and correct observation will by itself make us useful nurses, but that without it, we shall be useless with all our devotion.

-Florence Nightingale

The ability to concentrate or focus is the most intuitively recognized, essential skill for responding effectively in a high-stress environment like an emergency medical situation. Performance expert Dr. Robert Nideffer (1978) said this about concentration and attention:

> *It's the ability to control attention under pressure and in response to changing demands that separates the average person from the super performer.*

This observation has been supported by the work of Dr. Joan Vickers (2016) and others in what has been called 'quiet eye training.' Research has shown differences between highly skilled and lesser skilled athletes as to where they focus in critical decision moments (Wood & Wilson, 2016). Similar findings are emerging in relation to the eye gaze and location of the focus of highly experienced surgeons compared to less experienced surgeons and that quiet eye training can improve performance (Harvey et al., 2014; Causer et al., 2014). The same is true for nurses, where eye-tracking of focus was related to recognizing clinical signs and subsequent decision-making (Anton et al., 2023). Performance researchers (Janelle & Hatfield, 2008) summarize the importance of focus this way:

Simply stated, the most critical factor in high-level performance is attention to the right thing at the right time.

Concentration is perhaps the least understood and trained skill. Knowing that it's essential to concentrate during a nursing emergency is very different from knowing how to do so.

The brain has incredible capability. For example, read the following:

THE BRIAN IS TRLUY AMZAING AND CAN OFETN QUCIKLY SOVLE PRBOELMS AND SEEM TO MAKE SNESE OUT OF NOHTNIG.WTIH JUST MNIMIAL CUES, LIKE THE FISRT AND LSAT LEETTR OF A WROD BEING IN PALCE, THE BRAIN CAN CRORETCLY FILL IN THE RSET. THIS IS BCEAUSE WE DO NOT RAED EACH LEETTR, BUT THE WROD AS A WHOLE STERSS CAN RELLAY FOUL UP THIS ABIILTY, HWOVEER .THE BRIAN IS TRLUY AMZAING

It's remarkable that we can make sense out of such scrambled and minimal information, but we can. Of course, this is often the very nature of a medical emergency. You encounter minimal or confusing information or inconsistent symptoms, and you must quickly understand their meaning and significance in critical and chaotic situations.

When the emergency response team arrives, and staff starts shouting all kinds of information, what really matters? Being able to pick out the relevant details is crucial to making sure your patient has an optimal outcome.

While the brain can be brilliant in function, it's also sensitive to disruption by stress. We didn't always understand this. Stress effects on World War II combatants at Normandy were such that soldiers at that time were (unfortunately and incorrectly) characterized as 'slow-witted' because of their slowness in comprehending orders (Driskell et al., 2006). They also exhibited memory defects, as demonstrated by an inconsistent ability to relay orders. In retrospect, and with the advances in our understanding of stress and post-traumatic stress, it is easy to see why these soldiers appeared slow or 'stupid' when mortars and gunfire were raining down on them.

More recent studies (Lieberman et al., 2005) on the effects of stress on performance were conducted during combat simulations involving U.S. Army Rangers and BUD/S (Basic Underwater Demolition/SEAL) trainees. Compared to pre-stress levels, the studies found decrements in vigilance, reaction time, memory, and logical reasoning under stress.

Stress can also create a 'Jangle Effect,' which is that stress creates difficulty with some forms of reasoning (Murray, 2004). This is especially true for verbal problem-solving. Stress affects our internal dialogue (thinking that feels like 'talking to ourselves'). And unfortunately, it's this internal dialogue which we use to analyze and solve problems.

Considerable research shows that stress can produce a variety of negative effects on cognition (Kavanaugh, 2005). Stress can lead to:

➢ Reduced ability to analyze complex situations
➢ Reduced ability to manipulate information
➢ Making decisions on incomplete information
➢ Failing to consider a range of alternatives
➢ Ignoring long-term consequences of proposed solutions
➢ Oversimplifying assumptions and requiring more time to reach a solution

Group Think

Teamwork and high-performance teams are becoming more and more a part of healthcare delivery (Jain, 2007) and especially in emergency situations. The quality of teamwork determines outcomes (Salas et al, 2008), and the integration of individual performance remains an important factor in the quality of team function and success (Fernandez et al., 2008).

Of particular importance at the team level in emergency care is the phenomenon of stress-based 'Group Think' (first discussed by Janis in 1973). Group Think is a distortion of the creative potential for group problem-solving that occurs when stress is not managed. The characteristics which degrade the potential synergy of a team under stress include:

- An illusion of invincibility creates excessive optimism leading to extreme risks
- Unquestioned belief in the group's morality
- Stereotyped views of the challenge and underestimation of the threat
- Group members ignoring important information
- Direct pressure on members to conform, especially those who express a counterview

Stress can also affect cognition by mental stalls, where cognitive processes fail at one or more of several points in thinking through a response in a crisis. Disruption can occur at any or all phases of analyzing a crisis (much like that of situational awareness):

- ➢ The Perception Phase- you're not paying attention, or you don't see the problem.
- ➢ The Analysis/Evaluation Phase- you cannot identify the problem, or you misinterpret the significance.
- ➢ The Strategy Formulation Phase- your decision-making is absent or disrupted by stress.
- ➢ The Motor Initiation Phase- stress causes you to "freeze" or slows your actions.

Concentration is an essential skill for optimal response in any emergency nursing situation.

Concentration is the ability to direct and maintain your thoughts and attention. Consider the following. Are these statements true or false?

- ➢ Concentration is an automatic reflex.
- ➢ Concentration cannot be learned.

> Because we concentrate every day, practice is not needed.

> Concentration requires little energy.

> Our level of concentration always fits the situation.

All of the above statements are false.

The true statements would read this way. The ability to concentrate is not fully automatic. Concentration can be and needs to be trained. Daily use does not create the type of intense concentration needed in emergency nursing situations. Concentration takes a great deal of energy and can be quite tiring. There is often a mismatch between the degree of concentration needed in a situation and one's ability to engage in it.

Excellence in concentration is a requirement for safe and successful action in emergency situations because sub-optimal concentration leads to sub-optimal performance and poor outcomes. Perry (2005) notes that once a skill is well-learned or automated, it requires less conscious attention. However, pressure can shift attention away from relevant information or cues and interfere with learned behavior. This is when 'choking' (the inability to respond usefully) can occur.

When you hear a colleague say, "That was a stupid mistake," "Did that really happen?" or "I never saw it coming," what is really being described is a lapse in attention and concentration. Nurses are not stupid (so "stupid mistakes" don't occur), but the ability to adequately control attention and concentration can be an issue. This is especially true with difficult patients or on protracted and tiring shifts.

How's your Focus?

Here is a brief informal exercise to test your concentration and feel the 'work' of concentrating. Note the words SMALL and LARGE written in the columns below. Beginning at the top of the first column, time yourself as you read (aloud) down the list of words as fast as you can. Then immediately proceed to the second column, then the third, fourth, and fifth until you reach the last word at the bottom of the last column. Note your time. Ready. Go!

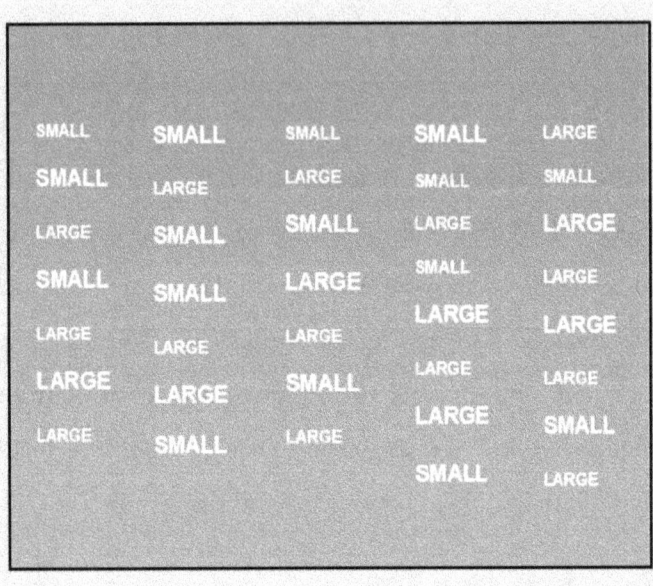

How long did it take you?

Now do the same thing with the next block of words. But this time, do not read what the word says, but say whether it's printed in large or small font. For example, you would read Large as large, but Large as small; and Small as large and Small as small. .

Ready. Go!

SMALL	SMALL	SMALL	SMALL	LARGE
SMALL	LARGE	LARGE	SMALL	SMALL
LARGE	SMALL	SMALL	LARGE	LARGE
SMALL	SMALL	LARGE	SMALL	LARGE
LARGE	LARGE	LARGE	LARGE	LARGE
LARGE	LARGE	SMALL	LARGE	LARGE
LARGE	SMALL	LARGE	LARGE	SMALL
			SMALL	LARGE

How long did it take you this time?

You were probably slower (and made more mistakes) the second time as you had to concentrate harder. In fact, you probably felt your brain working at separating out the word cues from the size cues, a process much slower than just reading the words. This is based on the famous 'Stroop Test,' which demonstrates how difficult it can be to filter out irrelevant information. The obvious conclusion is that complex or unfamiliar tasks impair (slow) cognitive responding.

Another Test of Your Ability to Focus

We have another informal concentration exercise for you located in Appendix I. This is from one of the pioneers in sport psychology, Dr. Dorothy Harris of Penn State University. Don't turn to the appendix yet. When you do, you will find a grid with randomly distributed numbers from 00 to 99. Start by finding the 00 and crossing out consecutive numbers (from 00 to 99; that is 00, 01, 02…09, 10, 11…) as far and as quickly as you can in one minute.

Now, turn to Appendix I and…Go!

How high did you get in one minute? There is no hard and fast data on this, but generally, high-level performers score in the mid to upper twenties. When I (MA) taught a sport psychology class at a college, I often had much of the football team in my class (looking for an easy A, I assume). They typically scored in the high teens to low twenties; the highest score, in my experience, was turned in by a professional soccer goalkeeper who was able to find thirty-five numbers in one minute.

If you scored less than this, don't be concerned. This doesn't mean that you are deficient at concentrating; it simply means that you probably don't practice and use it the way that athletes do. More importantly, the purpose of the drill was to show concentration is not automatic and that there is always room for improvement.

There are some aspects to concentration and attention that are important to understand in order to maximize your response in high-stress situations. The first is the breadth or width of concentration, attention, or awareness. Attention can be broad; that is, it can have a wide perspective, or it can have a narrow and tight focus. Just as with arousal, different tasks require or can tolerate different breadths of attention. Consider the sports skills and activities below and decide whether each requires a broad/wide-range focus or a pinpoint/narrow focus. Write the skill under the appropriate column.

OPTIMAL BREADTH OF ATTENTION IN SPORTS

Hockey Goalkeeping
Archery
Diving
Basketball Defense
Basketball Free-Throw

Pinpoint/Narrow   Broad/Wide-Range

The following charts suggests where the skills might be placed.

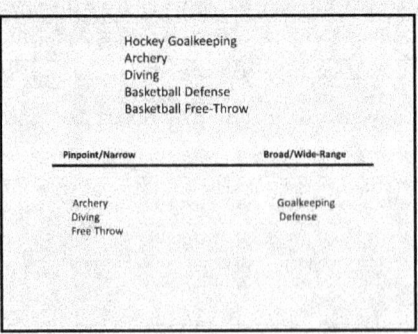

Clearly, archery or putting requires a much narrower focus (on the bullseye or hole) than watching the court in basketball defense, which requires scanning the court to read the play. Of course, many sports activities require the ability to shift attention from narrow to broad, broad to narrow, and back and forth. A quarterback must first broadly read the defense, survey what is happening on the field, and then zoom in on his targeted receiver, all while players move about. A goalkeeper needs to survey the entire ice, then focus on the attacking player while watching his defensemen and opposing players.

Now, let's do the same drill with the medical emergency skills listed here. Place them where they should be:

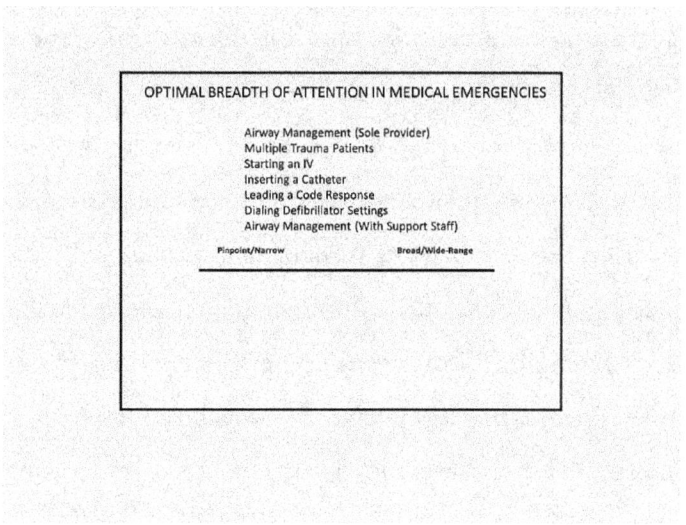

Here are some suggestions on where these skills might fit.

OPTIMAL BREADTH OF ATTENTION IN MEDICAL EMERGENCIES

Airway Management (Sole Provider)
Multiple Trauma Patients
Starting an IV
Inserting a Catheter
Leading a Code Response
Dialing Defibrillator Settings
Airway Management (With Support Staff)

Pinpoint/Narrow	Broad/Wide-Range
Solo Airway	Multiple Trauma
Staring an IV	Leading a Code
Inserting a Catheter	Team Airway Management
Dialing Defibrillator Settings	

Again, this is not a prescription for concentration in these circumstances, but to help you consider the relationship between certain skills and types of concentration. In medical emergencies, too, many situations require the ability to shift attention from broad to narrow or narrow to broad, and back again. Starting an IV requires a different focus than leading a code and assessing if all the required personnel and supplies are present. Assuring a match of concentration to the requirements of the situation is the key to enhancing performance.

Locus of Focus

The other aspect of attention and concentration is called locus of focus, which refers to the location of your focus. Is your attention focused internally (inside yourself, such as thoughts, feelings, physical sensations) or externally (outside yourself on what is going on around you)?

Most often, it's best to be externally focused - to be aware of what is going on around you during a medical emergency. It would inhibit your responding properly if you were internally focused - being distracted by anxiety, discomforts, or other thoughts and sensations - when you should be processing the events of the emergency. However, there are times when it's useful to be internally focused; being aware of what is going on within your body and in your thinking such as assessing your fatigue levels, recognizing when you need to take a break, or knowing if you need to increase your pace or actions.

So, as noted, it's usually best to be externally focused, especially when you need to receive information or orders. It's also important when you need to assess how others are doing. Being able to observe if and when those on your team are struggling or need a break can help the rest of the team function better. External focus also helps when you need to distract yourself from discomfort or fatigue to continue functioning.

Intuition

The role of intuition in decision making and especially in emergencies is an important and fascinating topic. Tuition often seems to be a somewhat mystical and inexplicable process that allows us to make decision and choices without seeming to 'think about it.' In fact, some work suggests individuals do not always follow a logical decision process, especially in critical situations.

Indeed, the components and skills called 'intuition' in various situations, including medical emergencies, are not magical processes or rare abilities. Intuition has been described (Zimmerman, 2008) as a

> "… *package of cues, perceptual processes, situation recognition and action-choice evaluations…*" which "*can be deconstructed, evaluated, and enhanced, giving understanding to the previously mysterious outcomes attributed to intuition.*"

Intuition may be much like System I responses that are sensed, but are unable to initially be verbalized. Further, those individuals who successfully use intuition are often well-experienced with the situations in which decisions are made or skills needed. It is also likely related to what has been called Recognition Primed Decision-Making (RPDM) which is based on experience that experts have amassed that allows them to quickly recognize and analyze the essential features of a situation (Klein, 2003; Graham, 2010). Integrating psychological and physical skills training (and repeated training) can enhance the components and skills that are often called intuition.

Enhancing Attention and Concentration

As with the discussion of sympathetic arousal and quality of performance, the point here is to begin to think about what type of attention you need for different skills and tasks during a medical emergency. Are you engaged in the appropriate type and can you adjust focus as needed? There are three dimensions to concentration and three related questions to ask yourself about the quality of your attention and concentration:

Intensity: Can I concentrate hard enough?

Duration: Can I concentrate long enough?

Flexibility: Can I shift attention as needed?

If you cannot answer an emphatic 'Yes' to each of these, you will benefit from training your concentration and attention skills. This is essential, not only for excelling in performance, but also for avoiding performance decrements and mistakes.

There are a variety of ways to attempt to increase the effectiveness of concentration. As a basis, Perry (2005) reports that gaining an optimal level of arousal leads to optimal attention skills. So once again, being able to create your O-ZONE is an important foundational skill. Actual training techniques for enhanced concentration range from simple exercises to rather involved computer-driven training. Some simpler suggestions are described in this next section.

Test, Test, Test

It has been said that "remembering enhances remembering," and now research confirms this. Testing and challenging yourself and/or others increases retention of material that is learned. The research compared the effects of repeatedly studying material to repeatedly testing the material. At the conclusion of training, all individuals scored close to 100% on this test of memory skill. But one week later, the repeated study group was able to produce only about 35% of the answers correctly, while the group that was repeatedly tested had 80% accuracy in their responses (Price, 2008).

Video Games

Fortunately, there is a readily accessible and affordable alternative to expensive computer-driven concentration training; computer and video games. Research on video games (Dingfelder, 2007; Green et al., 2006) shows that regular players of certain games are exceptionally fast at visual searches, at monitoring a larger field of vision (attending to the center of their vision and the periphery simultaneously), were more flexible in their attention, and excel at target location. While it is known that training using search simulations can improve visual attention in air traffic controllers and fighter pilots, it's not clear if it transfers to other situations.

Not all video games present the necessary cognitive challenges to build concentration and perceptual strengths, however. You need to give some thought as to whether the video game you choose to play challenges the types of skills that will be valuable in an emergency situation.

NASA looked at training astronauts in regulating their physiology as a way to control hazardous operator states, such as distracted attention (Prinzel, Pope & Freeman, 2001). To make it more interesting, NASA attempted to link playing video games to desired states of attention. Games were made accessible to the astronaut when he was in a desirable state of alertness (the games only turned on when the astronaut was in the target emotional/ psychological/ physiological state). This led to the astronaut's awareness of such optimal states being strengthened and the techniques to achieve such states being practiced more regularly.

Attention-Fixation Training

Attention-Fixation Training is an even simpler and more readily accessible technique that can help train concentration. You begin by sitting in a quiet place and choosing an object, usually medically related like your stethoscope, and concentrating on it. The idea is to learn to focus solely on the object and nothing else.

Notice its shine, the way it reflects light or color, and any scuffs or scratches. Hold only these instrument-related thoughts in your mind. Try to maintain this focus initially for fifteen to thirty seconds.

The degree to which you can do this is a measure of your attentional discipline. If you find thoughts entering your awareness unrelated to your stethoscope - "Why am I doing this stupid crap," "I have other priorities," "I'm bored…" know that they represent thought drifting, distractibility, and decreased attentional discipline. When it happens, and it will, don't get frustrated. Simply bring your focus back on the object.

Slowly increase the concentration-time to about two minutes. Once you have reached this sustained attentional goal, begin to introduce distractions. You might stream music at a low volume and see if you can ignore the music and maintain your attention on your stethoscope. We like using a talk radio program or podcast as a distraction with the goal of ignoring and being oblivious to the discussion being broadcast when you are focusing on your target object. With a strong focus on your stethoscope, you should have no idea what was said in the discussion.

When you're able to maintain focus successfully at a low volume, you should make the distraction more prominent, a bit louder, or more noticeable. Again, repeat this procedure until your focus seems solid, and then increase the distraction again. Continue to increase the distraction as your concentration skills improve.

Use sounds from a real-world setting in your concentration training. Focus on your stethoscope while listening to tapes of sirens, shouts, or sounds from codes. By training with sounds that mimic the type of settings in which you actually function, you more quickly transfer your skills to real-life situations. Record some old Gray's Anatomy or "ER" episodes of dramatized crises and play them in the background. We're not saying the shows were completely accurate (or realistic), but the sounds are probably similar to the sounds of your own hospital setting.

Train in the real world. It is important to move your practice to 'live' settings and to train with the goal of maximizing transfer to the real world. Create an opportunity for concentration training in the ED, ICU, or on the clinical floors. Obviously, this is not an excuse to sit at your workstation for large periods of time and ignore the world and then tell your boss you were practicing concentrating. However, take a few minutes each week or even daily to practice. Maybe you can do it at the start of your shift or immediately after lunch before you get back into the workflow.

Finally, broaden and alternate the distraction from narrow to broad. Using a similar approach as that to train your narrow focus as above, begin shifting your attention from the focus object to the distraction. For example, when using music as a distraction, shift your attention to listening to it and ignore the focus object (while still looking at it). Then become aware of and focus on other sounds and objects or activity in station; then shift back to the original focus object. Remember, most emergency situations will require flexibility in your focus. Continue to train, shifting your focus until it becomes a habit. It is an easy thing to practice, and the skill and benefits develop quickly.

To summarize: the above technique trains attention to strengthen and focus, which is often the hardest thing to do in highly charged, distracting situations. But as noted before, too much narrowing can also occur, as in tunnel vision and auditory exclusion. The above exercise can be used to train attention flexibility and broad situational awareness, as well.

Music Compartmentalization

Music compartmentalization involves listening to your favorite music in a different way. When listening to favorite songs, try to notice melody lines or instrumental riffs you were not aware of before. Try to focus away from the words or main melody and focus on the bass or saxophone. See if you can pick out the bass line or drum rhythms and follow them while ignoring the melody or words on which you usually focus. Move back and forth between a narrow, intense focus to a broad comprehensive one of all the sounds you are hearing.

Driving Scans

Driving in your car provides another excellent opportunity to practice strengthening your concentration and situational awareness. While driving, you can practice regular scanning of the environment (something you should be doing anyway).

That is, briefly, intermittently, but consistently shift attention from the car in front of you to other aspects of the road and your drive; become aware of the car behind you, the one to the side, traffic flow, sidewalk activity, and pedestrian behavior. You can do the same procedure with auditory awareness. Scan particularly for potential hazards as you narrow and broaden your attention and develop scanning as a habit.

VII. Mental Scans: Performance Enhancing Mental Imagery & Performance

Differences in skill acquisition in favor of mental rehearsal are important, especially when this technique is used in the teaching of life-saving skills such as cardio-pulmonary resuscitation and the use of defibrillation.

Fountaki et al., 2021

Mental imagery, also called mental practice, is a natural process that can be one of the most powerful psychological skills for enhancing performance in emergency medical situations. You probably already engage in mental imagery quite regularly when you anticipate your involvement in any situation, including patient encounters, presentations when teaching other nurses, or what lies ahead of you on a night shift.

Although the use of mental performance imagery has a long history in human performance enhancement, it is perhaps best known and most widely used in high-level athletic competition. Dr. Shane Murphy, former head of psychological training for the United States Olympic Committee says (2005):

Imagery…is the most important of the mental skills required for winning the mind game in sports.

Performance Enhancing Mental Imagery (PEMI)

Remsberg (1986) may have been one of the first to discuss imagery in high-stress situations. He called it 'crisis rehearsal,' which was a good idea, but perhaps not the best term, since it is not the crisis, but the response to the crisis that should be the focus of imagery training. In addition to sports, the use of imagery has been recognized as useful in many critical situations, including medical emergencies (Asken, 1993, Asken 2020) and military, police, and surgical crises (Murray, 2004; Asken, 2005; Asken et al., 2009, Asken & Yang, 2021).

Imagery practice was originally defined as the symbolic rehearsal of a motor skill in the absence of any gross muscular movement (Richardson, 1969). PEMI, as we will refer to it, is the use of your imagination to improve performance and the specific skills needed in emergency medical situations. Consider it a mental practice and mental rehearsal of skills you will use to save a life.

Uses for Performance-Enhancing Mental Imagery

PEMI can be used to enhance performance in several ways, including:

- Improving cognitive and motor skills
- Analyzing and correcting errors
- Simulating situations
- Preparing for specific situations
- Gaining 'experience'
- Maintaining skills
- Enhancing confidence

PEMI can be used to improve cognitive and motor skills. It can complement and enhance training of emergency response skills, such as assessment, establishing an airway, and even personal and team interaction skills. Hall (2002) has written an excellent article on the neurophysiologic basis of mental imagery and its application to training surgical skills. He reports potential benefit for both motor and cognitive skills and states:

Surgical educators should appreciate that imagery practice is an important component of skill development.

Goodspeed and Lee (2007) strongly endorse the use of 'visualization' to prepare for and enhance performance during a medical or surgical procedure. They state that visualizing a medical procedure is the next best thing to doing it. They go on to say:

The better you can visualize the procedure, the better you'll perform it that first time, regardless of the circumstances.

Sanders and his colleagues (2008) note that surgeons (and athletes) frequently use mental imagery in preparing to perform. PEMI has been suggested as an important component of mental preparation for surgeons prior to a procedure (Asken et al., 2020).

Mental imagery has been suggested as a useful technique to help in patient care (Santos, 2016). Others have seen it as a way to reduces nurses' stress and even promote development as graduate nurses (Contrades, 1991; Boehm & Tse, 2013).

Related to general nursing skills, there is some research on mental imagery with nurses to improve training in intramuscular injections, donning and doffing sterile gloves, and one-rescuer CPR, but with minimal impact (Doheny, 1993; Bucher, 1993; Bachman, 1990). However, research has shown nurses are capable of utilizing imagery and find it useful, are able to improve their imagery ability, find it reduces anxiety, and that it increases sense of well-being, quality of sleep, energy, and self-confidence (Bachman, 1990; Eaton & Evans, 1986; Stephens, 1992).

Studies by Ignacio and colleagues (2016; 2017) found variable results, but overall benefit in integrating mental rehearsal in training nurses to recognize signs of deterioration in patients. Combining mental rehearsal with training in the RAPIDS (Rescuing a Patient in Deteriorating Situations) technique, they found it was equivalent to training with the ABCDE mnemonic, but did not show a greater impact on reducing stress. While there are a number of problems with the design and content of these studies, interviews with nurse participants found a positive response to the mental rehearsal in a variety of ways. For example, nurses felt the mental imagery training helped in recall and use of the mnemonic (2017):

> *It puts the scenario in a story line, rather than just using the ABCDE, (it's) easier to visualize…it's like a retrieval tool… You must have knowledge before, then with mental rehearsal, you can use it to draw out the information that you have or you know.*

PEMI remains a technique of promise for maximizing nursing skills such as CPR and further research is ongoing (White, 2019).

PEMI can be particularly useful to you with skills that are sequenced, such as ACLS actions. By imaging the details of the algorithm, you not only 'practice' the procedures, but you can also check for any points of uncertainty or confusion regarding the appropriate next step. If you cannot complete the procedure smoothly in your imagery, you probably cannot execute it effectively in reality.

PEMI can be especially useful to you in the early stages of learning a new technique and can help reduce time needed to complete a learning curve (Hall, 2002). Not engaging in imagery may actually impair learning a simple motor task. However, modeling skills by an instructor or another person is more effective than performance imagery when first learning a skill (SooHoo et al., 2004). Other authors say that performance imagery for skill improvement can be effective for both novice and experienced individuals (Morris, Spittle & Watt, 2005).

It seems reasonable that some initial exposure to a nursing technique or situation is necessary, so that imagery can reflect reality and be imaged correctly. Without some experience, imagery will be entirely creative and quite possibly incorrect. Performance imagery is not performance fantasy! Reading about defibrillation as a nursing student would most likely not be enough exposure to practice PEMI. However, after watching a video or hands-on training, PEMI can help to quickly refine and solidify the skill.

Once PEMI techniques are mastered, they can have various applications. There is an interesting story (Moran, 1996) that shows the cross-over of imagery training from sports to other complex motor skills. PEMI is a common performance technique used by professional golfers. While pursuing another hobby, Master's champion Nick Faldo said this about his helicopter pilot training:

I took time off in the privacy of my room to spend ten minutes simulating in my mind how to land my helicopter. By the time the next lesson came around, I discovered not only was I an expert in landing it in theory, I could suddenly land it in reality, too. (p.209)

That PEMI is easy to use and can be used almost any time and anywhere is illustrated in another story (Murray 2004). Performance expert Ken Murray tells of meeting baseball great Mark McGwire. He approached McGwire, who was sitting by himself at a party, to inquire about skill development. When asked how often he practiced, McGwire's response was that he had just been sitting there knocking balls out of the park in his head until Murray had interrupted him.

An important recognition is that negative imagery, imagery of performance problems or failure, is also impactful, but in degrading the quality of performance. Negative imagery can reduce the quality of technical performance. Just as we will see when we examine negative thinking, the impact of negative imagery may be even more powerful than that of positive imagery (Murphy, 2005) and, so, is to be avoided.

PEMI has an important role in analyzing and correcting errors. In training, as well as in actual situations, you can use PEMI to review your sequence of actions and define points where you experienced uncertainty, confusion, and potential or actual mistakes. Then by imaging a more preferred or effective response, you can 'erase the old tape' of sub-optimal performance and errors and 'reprogram' or 'tape over' a more successful response that can be stored for later use. Failure to image correct and effective performance after mistakes leaves the residue of failure in your brain. This is especially useful in simulation training if you are not able to repeat an evolution and actually practice a corrected or improved technique.

PEMI can be used effectively to simulate a situation and prepare for a specific situation. It is used to rehearse situations that you might not have had an opportunity to practice in training. It can be used to anticipate and rehearse different approaches or conditions that might occur: missing items on the crash cart, simultaneous emergencies, or even the care of a celebrity with attendant media and entourage pressures. Granted, you can't imagine every possible scenario you will ever face, but you can imagine more variations than you can physically practice.

You can use PEMI to gain 'experience' with situations that can't be recreated easily or frequently either in physical simulation or live training. Murray (2004) discusses work that shows that survivability in air combat is greatly increased after a pilot's first five combat engagements. However, getting to or through the first five engagements for a pilot may take time and is certainly dangerous.

Anders Ericsson (2008), who spent years studying the nature of expertise, found that mastery in sports, arts, the sciences, and medicine takes thousands of hours and a specific type of practice, called deliberate practice, before world-class status can be achieved. PEMI can give you experience with a plan on how to handle your response when a code is called while you are monitoring a frail patient in the bathroom, dispensing time-bound critical medication, or when it occurs during the chaos of a shift change. You can't speed up time, but you can fill your time with more experiences through PEMI.

It is clear that experience can increase your confidence and competence in nursing skills, but as stated before, it is not clear how many practice sessions or simulations you will need (Hall, 2002; Barrett, 2006). Although PEMI is not the actual experience, it can substitute for the real thing when that specific training situation or actual situation is not available.

PEMI can help maintain your skills, or at least, slow their decay. As a powerful tool, you can use PEMI to keep skills fresh, it has been said that:

…even when you don't have the resources to actually practice a skill, positive mental imagery is a tool that those who are at the top of their game use to maintain and improve proficiency (Murray 2004).

The 'stale beer effect,' or atrophy of skills, was discussed earlier. Lammers et al., (2008) state that procedural skill decay, or the loss of some or all of the component skills necessary to perform a procedure after a period of non-use, has been well established in medical training.

Examples include airway management and CPR skills which can degrade in as little as two weeks to fourteen months. Even Advanced Life Support knowledge and skills of anesthesiologists diminished, such that only thirty of forty-seven achieved passing performance at six months post-training and also increased time to first defibrillation occurred (Wang, et al, 2008; Semeraro, et al., 2005). For nurses, the insertion of an inner cannula as part of a trache procedure and care may fade quickly as a skill, but might be maintained with the help of PEMI.

PEMI can be used to enhance your confidence. While enhanced confidence is often a result of experience and effective mental preparation for an emergency situation, it can be further improved more directly by imaging needed technical and emotional responses. Research shows that performance imagery can affect anxiety, motivation, and feelings of effectiveness.

And again, it can block unwanted negative imagery where feelings of confidence are decreased, and not just performance (Morris,et al., 2005).

Performance anxiety dreams are not an infrequent occurrence in high-achieving individuals. In academics, dreams of being late to class, having forgotten to do an assignment, inability to find a classroom, and having a pen malfunction, all occur. Such dreams may occur in nurses and other medical providers invested in bringing the best possible care to patients.

While such dreams are more uncomfortable than problematic, a form of imagery called Imagery Rehearsal Therapy may have promise for reducing such dreams. (Krakow, et al., 2001; Gibson, 2006). In short, imagery rehearsal treatment involves imagining different, more positive, or effective actions or endings to the dreams after they occur and while awake. The new action or endings are then rehearsed through imagery practice. The interested reader is encouraged to search out Krakow's and Gibson's work.

Enhancing Effectiveness of PEMI

While you probably already tend to engage in imagery to some degree, there are ways to make your imagery maximally effective. These include:

- Image using all of your senses.
- Use the best perspective.
- Image skills and actions correctly.
- Image in real time.
- Image problems, but also solutions.
- Use movement and kinesthetic imagery.
- Make your images vivid.

PEMI is sometimes called 'visualization,' (e.g. Goodspeed & Lee 2007). We don't like or recommend this term because it implies you image only what you 'see' or 'visualize' during an emergency situation. During an actual crisis, all of your senses are working, so the mental rehearsal with PEMI should include all of your sensory responses. It's crucial to experience:

- What you would See

- What you would Hear
- What you would Feel (both tactile sensations and emotional reactions)
- What you would Smell
- What you would Taste

Using all of your senses promotes the best transfer of imagery responses to the real situation.

Research has attempted to look at the effects of visual imagery (imagining what you see) versus kinesthetic imagery (imagining what you physically feel). While a conclusion is not clear, it seems that for performance, integrating kinesthetic imagery is crucial to maximizing the benefit of imagery training, if not preferable (Murphy, 2005).

Two other related factors that affect the impact of imagery training are the vividness and controllability of the images. The more vivid (intense, realistic) your image, the more effect it will have. Controlling the image, staying on the skill, maintaining its vividness, and the like, also affect the impact of imagery training.

Imagine This

Try the following: Sit in a comfortable chair, relax, and close your eyes. For each instruction below, imagine the scene for a few moments, then open your eyes, clear your thoughts, and move on to the next scene. Make each image as vivid as possible, maintain your focus, and try not to allow other thoughts to distract you. (You may want to have someone read the following instructions to you). If anything about this makes you uncomfortable, please discontinue doing this exercise and read on.

- In your mind's vision, SEE a patient being rolled onto a chest compression board.
- In your mind's audition, HEAR the commotion of others' actions; vitals, and details on the patient.
- In your mind's touch, FEEL the chest compression board as you help lift the patient, the coolness of the patient's skin.
- In your mind's emotion, FEEL a sense of confidence as you approach the patient's room to render aid.
- In your mind's olfaction, SMELL the odor of sanitizing agents used to clean the room.

> In your mind's gustation, TASTE a cool drink on your parched and hoarse throat after you successfully concluded your care.

This gives you an idea as to how to use PEMI in all of your senses. Substitute other situations related to your particular responsibilities as a way to practice and enhance imagery beyond just the visual.

This exercise, like all those suggested in this book, are only for informational and educational purposes. If any aspect of any exercise is uncomfortable for you, it is best not continue the exercise, but rather seek further expert opinion on its use and/ or training for you.

While PEMI is a psychological technique, it doesn't mean you have to be perfectly still or passive when practicing imagery. Just as the imagery should include all your senses, it's allowable and recommended to move in motions that mimic the skills and actions that you are imaging. You may have seen Olympic ice skaters, prior to performing, going through the motions of their routine with their eyes closed to mentally and physically execute their skills. While not performed in full force, these partial physical movements can help make imagery more vivid and enhance the kinesthetic effects.

PEMI can be enhanced by considering the best perspective for you to use. If you are comfortable, do the following. Close your eyes and imagine yourself performing a nursing (emergency) skill. Do this for three to five seconds and then open your eyes and consider what your imagery looks like. Was your imagery like watching yourself, or did you experience being in the actual situation?

These are at the main two perspectives for PEMI:

➤ The external or third-person perspective: You image the emergency situation as if watching yourself on a videotape, being outside yourself like watching on television or from a surgical gallery.

➤ The Internal or First-Person perspective: You imagine what you actually experience during an emergency situation, not watching yourself perform.

Below is an example of what imagery of adjusting an IV might look like from the external or third-person perspective.

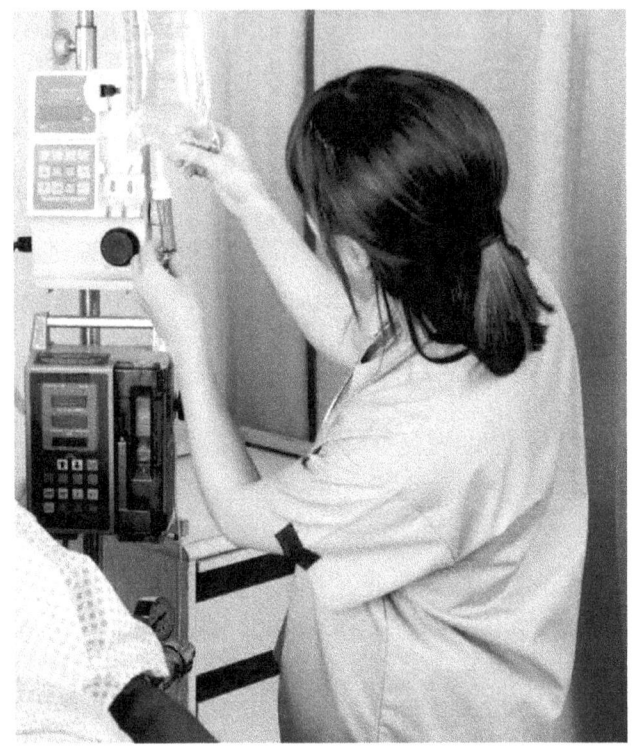

The following is an example of what you might see from the first-person perspective as you approach a patient's IV to make adjustments.

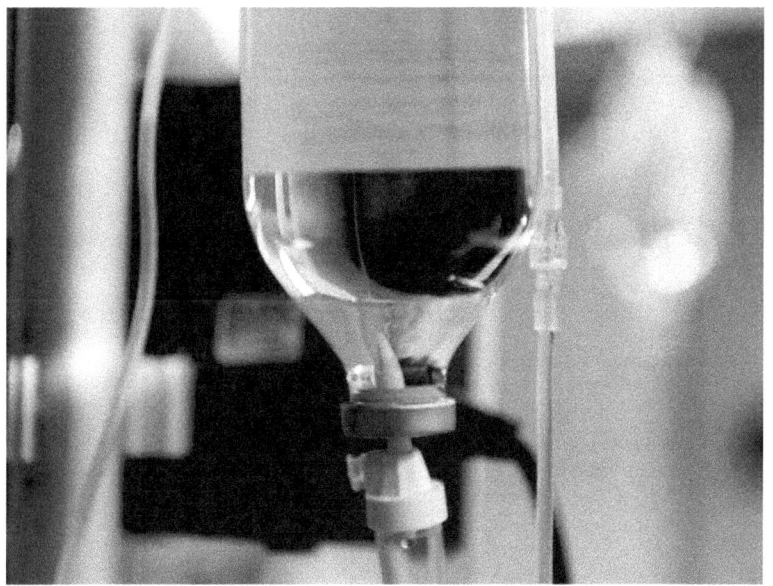

So, with performance-enhancing imagery in the third person or external perspective, you might see yourself or the scene from the distance as others might see you or as if observing yourself, like in the first picture. However, if you use first person or internal imagery, you would image a view like that you actually experience (see, hear, feel, etc.) in the situation as in the second photo above, rather than seeing yourself acting from the distance.

There are no firm conclusions about which perspective is best for enhancing performance. Initial reports indicated that elite athletes tended to use internal/first-person imagery; this made sense as this perspective is most like a real-life situation. However, later research found that the perspective used did not correlate with performance and being selected for elite teams. Further, other reports from Olympic athletes note that seventeen to thirty-five percent use internal/first-person imagery; thirty to thirty-nine percent use external/third person imagery, and thirty-four to forty-four percent use both (Morris, et al., 2005).

Personal experience in working with physicians, nurses, athletes, police, and military has engendered our preference for the internal/first person perspective. We believe the more realistic view is ultimately important. There is research that supports the use of this perspective in many elite-level athletes (Morris, Spittle & Watt, 2005).

However, since both perspectives can be effective, you should use the view that is most comfortable and works the best in terms of your performance. That being said, using both can also be effective. It makes sense that using the external perspective first, like watching a demonstration of the skill, is a good place to start. Then try imaging the execution of the skill operation from the internal perspective of actually being in it.

Practitioners of a technique called Neurolinguistic Programming (NLP) label the internal/first person view as the associated perspective and suggest it is effective in allowing the performer to 'step into' the imaged scenario and fully experience it. The external/third person view is called the dissociated perspective, and NLP suggests that it is very effective in observing and critiquing the quality of performance and gaining emotional distance (Andreas & Faulkner, 1994).

So you would use the associated (first-person) perspective when you really want to experience or be in the imagined scenario. You would use the dissociated (third-person) perspective to review how you are performing or when you want to have distance from the emotional impact of the imagined scenario. Perhaps the most important is to be sure to include kinesthetic and not just visual imagery.

PEMI is like physical practice, so practice skills and actions correctly. If you mentally rehearse a response sloppily or incorrectly, you will perform sloppily or incorrectly. There is an important lesson in the adage that "Practice does not make perfect; perfect practice makes perfect."

It's also our experience (or bias) that the focus of imagery should be on the 'process' rather than the 'outcome.' Since maximal performance comes from executing skills or plans as flawlessly as possible, this should be the focus of PEMI. Imaging the placement of the IV is more likely to result in successful positioning than imaging medicine infusing successfully. Dr. Mike Mahoney, a pioneer in sport psychology, often counseled that:

"If you focus on the process, the outcome takes care of itself."

Just as with physical practice, it may be useful to begin imaging a skill or action in slow-motion. However, ultimately the skill or action should be imaged in real time speed for the best effect.

It's useful and important for you to imagine difficult or even negative situations, such as uncontrolled bleeding, cardiac arrest, or a difficult intubation. Such negative or unanticipated events are often built into training scenarios as challenges. You should do the same with your imagery scenarios. The critical point is to never stop with the problem image but always go to a successful image of how that problem will be handled. In some potential situations, your options for intervention may be limited or not highly desirable; nonetheless, it is important to have imaged possible approaches for the situation, so you have prepared for an option.

There is an interesting parallel and important lessons about succeeding in surprising situations from research on driving skills (Mills, 2005). Most drivers are not trained for the unexpected. Because basic driving skills are so well-learned and because emergencies are rare, we become overconfident about our skills to handle them. Research shows that emergency attention skills do not improve automatically and, in fact, degrade without practice or reinforcement. We need to prepare and practice for the unexpected.

Just like physical training, PEMI should be practiced repeatedly to be effective.

As an additional approach to enhancing the effectiveness of imagery, you can use the acronym PETTLEP (Holmes & Collins, 2021):

P for Physical: Your imagery should be as similar to the actual physical skill as possible.

E for Environment: Your imagery should be practiced in the environment where the actual application will occur.

T for Task: Your attention during imagery should be focused on the same things as during actual execution of the skill.

T for timing: The effects of your imagery will be enhanced if the skill is imaged in real time, at the actual speed needed.

L for Learning: Your imagery should incorporate changes in feelings and techniques as your skill improves.

E for Emotion: Your imagery should include emotions associated with the event.

P for Perspective: You should use the perspective, external or internal, that works best for you.

An excellent approach to integrating physical and imagery practice is described by Loren Christensen in his book, The Mental Edge Revised (1999). He suggests a sequence of first imaging a skill, then doing the skill in pantomime. Finally, the skill should be performed in actuality. This type of sequence, IMAGE-PANTOMIME-PERFORM, nicely integrates the physical and psychological and can be applied to many training situations.

An interesting study showed the incremental value of PEMI in CPR training. It is important because it showed how psychological training can significantly improve emergency medical skills. While the study was completed with non-medical personnel, the relevance to medical professionals is clear.

Two concerns typically arise with CPR training in non-medical personnel:

1) Trained individuals are hesitant to use their skills.
2) Their retention of correct skills fades quickly over time.

The study by Starr (1987) incorporated performance imagery and psychological skills training with standard CPR training. The point of his study was to try to assess the effects of imagery and psychological skills-enhanced CPR training compared to standard CPR training on confidence and willingness to use learned skills. Additionally, the study assessed the drop-off incorrect responses in doing CPR that occurs over time. The results are summarized in the following:

PERFORMANCE OUTCOMES
OF
STANDARD VERSUS ENHANCED CPR TRAINING

Standard Vs Imagery Enhanced CPR Training

		6 Months	12 Months
Response Time (secs)	S-CPR	18.7	50.10
	IE-CPR	6.5	19.00
		6 Months	12 Months
Correct Responses (%)	S-CPR	75.56	53.33
	IE-CPR	93.33	88.00

The study compared performance between individuals trained by the standard CPR (S-CPR) training methods versus imagery-enhanced CPR (IE-CPR) that used psychological skills and imagery added to the traditional training.

First, the study measured how long it took individuals who were 'surprised' by an emergency situation to actually begin to administer CPR. The table shows that six months post-training, the imagery-enhanced group (IE-CPR) began emergency care in an average of only 6.5 seconds compared to an average response time of 18.7 seconds for those trained in the standard manner (S-CPR). When tested at twelve months post-training, the IE-CPR group again responded much faster at an average of 19.0 seconds compared to the S-CPR group that took an average of 50.1 seconds to respond.

The second part of the study looked at whether psychological skills training could help people to better remember how to do CPR correctly and effectively even when they hadn't used or practiced it for a long time. It was found that six months post-training, the IE-CPR group (psychologically trained) averaged 93.3 percent correct CPR skills compared to 75.6 percent correct for the S-CPR (standard training) group. At twelve months post-training, the IE-CPR group averaged 88.0 percent correct CPR skills compared to only 53.3 percent correct and effective skills for the S-CPR group. Thus, psychological skills training did help promote a faster response and help individuals maintain a higher quality of physical skills even over long periods of time.

Another relevant study was that by Fountouki et al. (2021), who looked at the impact of using mental rehearsal (PEMI) for training students in a nurse-assistant diploma program. The authors compared the performance of administering CPR or defibrillation in simulation between a control group and an experimental group coached in mental rehearsal. As can be seen from the data below, the students who received mental rehearsal training outperformed the control group on all outcome parameters of time to complete the CPR cycle, overall mistakes, CPR-related mistakes, and defibrillation-related mistakes.

Impact of Using Mental Rehearsal to Train Nursing Students in CPR Skills

	Time to Complete CPR (mins)	Overall Mistakes	CPR Mistakes	Defibrillation Mistakes
Control	8.5	5.5	2.4	3.2
Imagery	6.2	4.2	1.5	2.6

How PEMI Works

You may be wondering how is it that just thinking about a skill can improve its execution? There are several mechanisms that explain how mental practice improves physical performance (Suinn, 1985). These are:

- PEMI has physiological correlates.
- PEMI reduces surprise and uncertainty.
- PEMI produces emotion and emotional control.

Advances in physiological monitoring have provided the most dramatic and convincing evidence of how and why PEMI is effective. There are several examples.

In early studies, when athletes were attached to biofeedback monitors and imaged a skill but did not move, very small electrical signals could nonetheless be detected in muscles of the same body parts involved when the skill is actually executed. This suggested that performance imagery strengthens the connections between the brain and the parts of the body involved in actually doing the skill.

This has been part of psychoneuromuscular theory and is commonly termed 'muscle memory.' When you practice a skill, you are increasing the link between the brain and the involved body parts by strengthening nerve connections. Like physical practice, imagery seems to 'grease' the neural tracts from the brain to the body. The more greased these tracts become through repetition, the faster nerve impulses travel, and the more quickly and accurately you respond.

Most of the early and now more recent research used EMG (electromyographic) feedback and has been well summarized by Morris et al., (2005). Work by Jacobson in the 1930's showed that mental imagery of forearm bends, biceps curl, sweeping, and rope climbing produced more muscle activity with imagery than was produced when the same muscles were at rest.

Jacobson also showed that when subjects were asked to *visualize* performing a biceps curl (just 'seeing' the curl), ocular activity increased. But when they were asked to *imagine* experiencing a biceps curl (which involved all of their senses to experience the motion), it was actual, localized biceps muscle activity that increased. (This is another reason to use the word 'imagery' rather than 'visualization' for mental practice).

Working with U.S. Olympic athletes Suinn (1980) demonstrated similar results. Electromyographic (EMG) readings were taken of the leg muscles of U.S. Olympic skiers who imaged their race while at rest. It was found that the electrical activity in their legs and the activation of the activity reflected their description of where they were on the mountain and ski course.

A related source of evidence is near-infrared spectroscopy (NIRS). NIRS shows that when a skill is imaged, blood flow is increased to the part of the body involved in that skill. NIRS allows measurements of oxygenation and hemodynamic parameters.

A study (Griffin & Cooper, 2006) was done using NIRS measurements while an individual either rehearsed (imaged) squeezing a ball or actually squeezed the ball. It was found that imaging the squeeze (but not actually squeezing the ball) resulted in increased blood flow in the wrist (carpi radialis muscle).

Perhaps the most interesting evidence is found in various forms of brain scans performed during imagery. The use of functional magnetic resonance imaging (fMRI) supports the theory of functional equivalence. This theory says that many of the same parts of the brain are activated when imagining a scene as when actually viewing a scene. Areas of the brain activated with actual practice or performance are also activated with imagery alone (Murphy, 2005).

The same mechanism, or functional equivalence, may be present for motor skills, as well (Ingvar & Philipson, 1997; Morris et al., 2005). Subjects were asked to either imagine or actually clench their hands into fists. It was found that both methods changed the blood flow in the motor areas of the brain that control such movements. Other researchers are reported to have measured cerebral blood flow when golfers of various handicap levels imaged a golf swing. With imagery, increases in blood flow were found in areas of the brain that are associated with motor control, execution of motor skills, action planning, and error detection.

Additionally, we can now document that imagery, and mental practice creates changes in the brain. Typically, there is less brain activation in doing the task over time and with practice. In the first twenty minutes of learning, many areas of the brain are active. With every ten minutes, brain activity decreases, with a total reduction of about 85% of activity after the first hour. Decreased activity can be seen in brain areas that problem-solve, control tasks, use working memory, and involve attentional control. However, perceptual and motor areas of the brain involved in making actual responses remain more activated (Hill & Schneider, 2006). Less "brain power" is needed once a skill is mastered.

Another mechanism that explains the effectiveness of PEMI is that it reduces surprise and uncertainty. W.E. Hicks conducted research in the 1950's that showed that uncertainty or unfamiliarity and multiple possible responses slow reaction time. He found that as response options increased from one to two, reaction time increased (slowed response) by fifty-eight percent (Grossman, 2005).

By having practiced various scenarios, at least mentally, the situations and your responses to them become familiar, thus reducing any surprise factor. You're able to process a situation quickly because you recognize it. Although surprise or inexperience might delay your response for only fractions of a second (as you interpret a situation and determine a course of action), this is time that can be crucial in a medical emergency.

With imagery training, you respond more quickly and effectively because you recognize the situation (you have seen it in your imagery). It reduces the surprise, disbelief, and the typical and ubiquitous "Oh, Shit!" or "What do I do now?" reactions that delay effective responses in new and surprising situations.

PEMI has been likened to a "map app" on your phone. If you have a map app already installed, you enter the address, and off you go. However, if you don't have an app, you have to first go to an app store, peruse the choices, make a choice, download the app, and then enter the address. PEMI is like pre-loading your brain with apps or templates that help speed your actions at critical times.

Pattern Recognition is important for quick thought and action. It involves instantly evaluating the emerging pattern of an event by comparing it with a mental model. This mental model is typically developed by training and/or experience (Rahman, 2007), including proper PEMI training.

Pattern recognition abilities can be limiting, however. Without flexibility or broad training, patterns available to us can inhibit or misdirect our responses. For example, you can say the alphabet quickly and flawlessly when progressing forward from A to Z. But how smooth are you at saying it backwards from Z to A? Even though it's the same letters we have said and seen thousands of times, we learned them in a sequence that limits our reciting them backwards.

Thus, it is essential that you train and practice your actions in varied and changing conditions. PEMI can expand these variations and consequently expand your library of patterns and inputs to be used in recognition reactions. It can reduce negative anticipation and fill the time before an emergency situation with more productive anticipation.

Lastly, PEMI is effective because it not only trains and rehearses the skills of an emergency situation, it also produces emotions, and this can help mitigate emotional response in a real situation. Since imagery can produce physical changes in the body (muscle activity and brain-blood flow), as well as, autonomic changes (heart rate, skin temperature, and skin-blood flow), it can help you anticipate and learn to control these responses (Descahumes-Molinaro et al.,1992; Guillot,

2004). PEMI provides for practice of emotions found in high-stress situations and the focus and control needed in emotionally-charged ones. Rehearsal of these situations reduces their emotional impact.

PEMI is effective in helping individuals cope with feelings of increased sympathetic arousal. There are different forms of imagery that have different effects (Cummings et al., 2007). These include:

- Mastery Imagery: used to feel confident and in control
- Psyching-up Imagery: used to increase performance arousal
- Anxiety Imagery: used to create uncomfortable feelings
- Relaxation Imagery: used to produce calmness
- Coping Imagery: used to create feelings of being able to handle higher arousal

There is no definitive answer as to how much or how often you should practice imagery for maximum performance. Among Olympic athletes (Murphy, 2005), twenty percent use imagery every day, and forty percent use it three to five days per week. Timewise, there is some suggestion that to obtain the best results, you should practice imagery for either a period of one to three minutes or ten to fifteen minutes (Morris, et al., 2005). How much time and how often you need to practice imagery will depend on many personal factors, but you will come to know what works best for you and how to design your imagery routines.

Cautions in the Use of PEMI

There are some cautions associated with the use of imagery of which you should be aware. First, remember that PEMI is not as effective as physical practice. However, combining imagery and physical training can transfer well to overall performance.

As discussed previously, you will need some 'hands-on' experience with the skills or situations you want to image to achieve the best effect. Actual exposure and initial practice is best for this, although it can be approximated by vivid descriptions from instructors. PEMI must be based on the realities of the skills and situations, not solely on your assumptions and guesses about them. Remember that research suggests (Soohoo et al., 2004) that modeling of skills by others/experts was more effective than mental imagery for acquisition in the initial learning of motor skills.

Although nurses may vary in their ability to image, this should not be seen as a deficit or a problem. Almost everyone can generate imagery, though there are differences in how easily and effectively it can be done (Murphy, 2005). PEMI can be enhanced with practice, especially when you describe in detail what you're experiencing through your senses and by using vivid and highly descriptive words in the images. Eaton et al. (1986) found they could enhance imagery ability in nursing students through the use of imagery exercises. But even if you are not an effective imager, don't be discouraged, for there are other mental skills as described here that can elevate your performance.

Remember that imagery can cause anxiety, although this really reflects untrained imagery or inadequate practice. For example, this could occur when the psychologically undisciplined mind engages in images of failure or when you don't confront the stressful situation in imagery often enough (inadequate practice) to reduce the anxiety. The point of imagery training is to provide control and focus to promote quality and successful performance.

Another caution is that imagery may be distracting, meaning that it may consist of irrelevant actions or details. An example might be experiencing intrusive images of your plans for the evening while still engaged in an emergency situation. Again, this is more likely to represent untrained or undisciplined imagery. Trained imagery should direct and keep attention on the critical aspects of a skill or situation.

While rare, it has been cautioned that imagery can lead to overconfidence (Cummings et al., 2006). PEMI may create feelings of confidence about performance that exceed actual ability. This is known as 'imagination inflation.' Be open to feedback about your performance to balance it with your images.

PEMI, like deep relaxations techniques, should be used cautiously or with guidance in individuals with a history of trauma, PTSD, or other significant mental health issues.

To summarize, keep in mind these key points about PEMI:
- ➤ It is not a substitute for scenario or other skills training.

- The key is to simultaneously integrate live training with imagery training.

- Effective PEMI requires some level of experience with the skill or situation through physical training, practice, and/or briefing. It is unlikely that realistic and relevant images of skill or operations can be fully developed without having had some engagement with actual situations.

- Using imagery within the context of trained psychological skills should actually reinforce the practice of all skills and the importance of constant appropriate vigilance.

Visuo-Motor Behavior Rehearsal (VMBR)

You can combine the above techniques into more structured and complex psychological training programs. For example, Suinn (1984) developed Visuo-Motor Behavior Rehearsal (VMBR), which combines relaxation and imagery techniques. It's been used extensively and effectively with athletes, and it has been used in training firefighters (Asken, 1993).

It's best to learn VMBR with an expert trainer in a structured manner. However, generally speaking, VMBR begins by creating a tranquil state through relaxation techniques and unique relaxation cue word or phrase. Then the relaxation cue word is 'switched off' and imagery of past successes is experienced, and also the performance of a specific skill or situation to be enhanced is 'switched on.' This process is alternated until the individual can go through the phases alone and quickly to prepare for a challenge.

Suinn used VMBR to help U.S. Olympic skiers prepare for competition by getting into a relaxed state and then skiing the race mentally while reviewing critical points on the mentally imaged course and the strategies to handle them. The technique was used with firefighters to prepare for building searches, entrapments, and other high-risk situations (Asken, 1993).

Stress Inoculation Training (SIT)

Stress Inoculation Training (SIT) is a multi-faceted approach to mastering stress in difficult situations (Meichenbaum, 1976). SIT builds resistance to specific stressful situations and integrates well with simulation exercises. As mentioned, when discussing VMBR, the initial stress inoculation training typically needs the assistance of a psychologist skilled in this technique.

There are three phases to stress inoculation training. The first phase is Cognitive Preparation, during which the rationale and overview of SIT is presented and the problem, challenge, or stressful situation is analyzed. During Skill Acquisition and Rehearsal, specific arousal control skills, such as relaxation training and self-talk, are learned and practiced. The last phase is Application, the implementation of the skills.

There are four steps to applying SIT to master stressful situations:

- Preparation for Provocation: is where you prepare mentally for the event and review the philosophy and strategy for meeting it.
- Impact and Confrontation: is where you prepare for the way the event is likely to affect you and summon your practiced skills.

- ➢ Coping and Arousal: is the actual application of the arousal control skills and SIT training to the challenge when it occurs.

- ➢ Review and Adjustment: this is where you review the process for what worked and what did not for behaviorally and emotionally managing the event. You make adjustments and practice them to prepare for the next situation.

Simulation training is an excellent opportunity to test out this process. It allows you to anticipate a situation, practice responses to it, apply those responses, and review your performance. While the above example deals with controlling yourself and remaining calm, you can also use VMBR and SIT to prepare for situations where you might need to take more forceful action. This may include restraining a combative patient or participating in de-escalation with other members of the team to control a psychotic patient.

Thompson & McCreary (2006) have outlined three specific goals for SIT and reported three research-supported effects of its use. SIT can:

(1) Improve your performance by changing problematic or sub-optimal behavior in high-stress situations

(2) Improve your ability to self-regulate behavior and responses

(3) Increase your ability to cope with stressful situations

They describe studies that show that SIT can decrease performance anxiety, decrease state (situational) anxiety, and increase performance.

Remember, procedures such as VMBR and SIT typically need the guidance of an experienced trainer, at least initially. However, whatever the psychological approach, these techniques, as with all psychological skills, need to be practiced and adapted for safe and effective use in specific situations. In the end, these arousal control techniques can help you develop greater control over physical and psychological responses experienced in emergency situations and ultimately optimize your performance.

VIII. Mental Prescriptions: Step-Up, Self-Talk and Performance

Words are very powerful. They can either inspire you to greatness or make you feel like crap. This is why it's best to choose the words you hear and the principles you believe. After all, we are all given a choice every day: to wallow in self-pity or push ourselves to achieve great things despite our imperfections.

-Nurse Buff

In few other endeavors are cognitive skills as critical to performance as in medical emergencies. How and what you think has a profound effect on your performance at all times, but especially in high stress situations. Cognitive scientists have elucidated relationships between perception, cognition, and performance. This work and the performance applications of cognitive therapy techniques have shown that our thoughts have a strong effect on our emotions, behavior and, therefore, the quality of our performance.

Self-Talk

You, like most people, probably experience thinking as 'talking to yourself.' While we often make jokes about people who walk around talking to themselves, all of us do it internally much of the time. (While there are some people who think predominantly in pictures, most of us experience thinking as having a conversation with ourselves). This is called *"self-talk"* and it is a powerful process that affects your behavior and a powerful tool to maximize your performance.

The importance of self-talk is recognized in emergency care (Fernandez et al., 2008) where it has been suggested that performance and decision-making are increased when training strategies teach to 'think about thinking.' Even in simulation, combining scenarios with strategies like 'thinking aloud' is seen as having merit (Bond et al., 2008). Performance expert Dr. Jim Afremow labels the nature of self-talk as either being your inner enemy (negative self-talk) or your inner ally (performance-enhancing self-talk). He asks "What channel is your self-talk on?"

There are several aspects of self-talk that are important to understand with regard to how it affects performance. They are that:

- Self-talk always occurs before you say anything, do anything, or feel any emotion.
- Self-talk is fast and subtle and though you are often unaware of it, it is there.
- The more well-practiced a skill, the quicker and "quieter" the self-talk.
- You can become aware of your self-talk.
- You can change your self-talk.
- Changing your self-talk can modify your response and performance.

The importance of self-talk is not surprising when you recognize the profound influence words have on us. Remember this adage: "The pen is mightier than the sword"? The emotional, behavioral, and performance impact of words is powerful, as any songwriter, advertising executive, salesperson, or attorney will attest.

The Nurse, Physician, Placebo and Performance

The story is told of a surgeon who would go on to become chief of surgery at a prestigious medical school, but in the 1950's he was a military surgeon in Korea working day and night tending to our country's wounded. He developed appendicitis himself and underwent surgery. With typical warrior spirit, he wanted to return to the operatory and get back to work only hours after his own procedure, but the pain was too great. He asked the nurse for a pain shot but was informed that he had reached his allowed limit. Unhappy with the answer, being a surgeon and an officer, he raised his voice and insisted (i.e. threatened) until he got his pain shot. Shortly thereafter, he returned to the OR for his shift, pain controlled. The next day he reviewed his medical record to find that he had not actually received any additional pain medicine in the shot, but merely normal saline. Desire and expectation are indeed powerful influences (Carey, 2004).

Other research highlights how much words and expectations can affect our responses and performance. For example, individuals were asked to rate the pleasantness or unpleasantness of an odor. In one case, the odor was labeled as 'cheese' and in the other, the *same* odor was labeled 'body odor.' The odor labeled as cheese was given an average rating of *negative* 0.10. The *same* odor was rated a *negative* 0.86 when labeled as body odor. Even when smelling clean air, the air labeled as body odor was rated a *negative* 0.40 !

Words form expectations and as anyone in medical care should know, expectations are powerful. One area where the power of expectation is clearly demonstrated is in the phenomenon of the placebo effect, as in the above story of the battle surgeon. While traditionally this was seen as a curiosity, nuisance or negative, Medicine is now starting to look at how and why the placebo is effective and how this effect might be harnessed for positive change.

Dramatic examples of the placebo response are found in what are called sham surgeries (Moseley et al. 2002). This is where a patient believes a surgical procedure was performed, but in actuality, at most, an incision was made but nothing else done. Especially with surgeries designed to reduce chronic pain, positive results and relief of pain are often found even with such sham procedures. Expectations are powerful.

The relationship of words to action is described in *Developing the Survival Attitude* (Duran, 1999):

But you should understand that a relationship between words and actions does exist and that words can have a direct positive or negative impact...

Another example of the power of words is seen in the use of the word 'if.' Such awareness can alter some aspects of the way we train and how we prepare ourselves. As alluded to earlier in the book, instead of practicing what to do *'if'* a situation occurs, preparation or training should focus on what to do *'when'* a situation occurs. The change suggests greater certainty and confidence.

A final example comes from Special Forces, but may be applicable to the special circumstances of medical emergencies, as well. Martin (2006) explains why the word 'try' is not part of the Special Forces vocabulary:

I did not say TRY. TRY is a WEAK WORD. In Special Forces we don't give you a mission and tell you to try. In Special Forces, you will be handed a mission that seems impossible and be told <u>DO YOUR BEST</u>. It may seem like a small change, but the implications are huge.

All this becomes important when we consider the role of self-talk in the performance of daily responsibilities and especially in high-stress situations. There are several areas where your self-talk and focus can be directed during a medical emergency. These include:

- Content totally unrelated to the emergency situation
- Content related to the general nature of the emergency situation
- Content related to encouragement or evaluation of efforts
- Content related to specific decisions and actions that need attention

Your thoughts and focus can be totally unrelated to the emergency at hand. You may be thinking about getting home, your hunger, or that you would rather be at the beach.

Your thoughts and focus might be on general aspects of the emergency situation. You may be thinking about whether the patient is young or old, whether the emergency response team arrived quickly or not, whether you know anyone on the team, etc.

Your thoughts and focus might be on encouragement or evaluation of your efforts. You may be thinking "Let's get at it," "Let's do our best," or "We're moving right along here."

Or, your thoughts and focus might be on the specific decisions that need to be made and actions that need to be taken. This is much like an instructor sitting on your shoulder and whispering (or yelling!) in your ear and talking you through what you should be doing in the emergency situation; what specific actions you should be taking. This is known as *"task-relevant instructional self-talk"* (Asken, 1993).

Which one of the above foci do you think will have the greatest positive impact on your performance?

The obvious answer is 'task-relevant instructional self-talk.' This is the only focus that can consistently enhance your performance and, therefore, your success. It is even more important than that of encouragement and pep talks since encouragement may have an effect on motivating you to do a good job, but it does not tell you *how* to do a good job. The famous Nike saying of 'Just Do It' is catchy and motivating, but fails to tell you *what* to do to act successfully.

Ericsson, (2008) in discussing the nature of expertise, reports that expert performers are able to report their thought processes and crucial aspects of an encounter. They know that telling themselves how to do a good job and exactly what to do is crucial to success.

We like to call developing and using task-relevant instructional self-talk as being able to **STEP-UP or STEPPING-UP** (**S**elf-**T**alk for **E**nhanced **P**erformance-**U**nder **P**ressure). As we said, being able to STEP-UP (or STEPPING-UP) is like having your instructor or mentor sitting on your shoulder and giving you specific instructions on what to do at each point in the code. This type of self-talk is often a series of short cues.

As an example, adapting recommendations for emergency care from Schaider et al. (2007), STEP-UP for an open ankle fracture might look like this:

- ➢ Emergency orthopedic consult or referral
- ➢ Remove contaminants
- ➢ Apply moist sterile dressing
- ➢ Assess tetanus immunity
- ➢ Antibiotics

STEP-UP for an animal bite might look like this:

- ➢ Wound irrigation
- ➢ Debridement
- ➢ Wound closure
- ➢ Antibiotics
- ➢ Extremity elevation
- ➢ Tetanus prophylaxis

While the STEP-UP statements do not contain all the details of actions that might be taken, they should allow you to keep a focus and be cues the interventions that are needed.

The use of task-related self-talk is important in that it also blocks your negative self-talk. When things are not going well it is easy to get into a negative thinking cycle, sometimes called 'Stinkin' Thinkin'.' We will discuss this more later. For now, realize that negative self-talk gets in the way of your performance; so avoid it. STEPPING-UP can help you achieve this goal.

There are several ways to train yourself to STEP-UP more effectively. These include:

- ➢ Relax or attain your optimal zone of nurtured excellence (O-ZONE).
- ➢ Encourage yourself.
- ➢ Encourage others.
- ➢ Monitor and change self-talk.
- ➢ Focus on actions and skills. Phrase self-instructions in the positive.

STEPPING-UP can be improved by first achieving your O-ZONE, as performance is maximized in this condition. Understand the level of arousal that works best for you and know how to create it. Use the techniques we discussed earlier to create your O-ZONE.

It is critical to *encourage yourself*. Believe that what you do is incredibly important, difficult, and skilled work. Using words like 'stupid' and 'idiot' to describe yourself (or others) when you make a mistake, or when things are not going well, is never appropriate or accurate and should be avoided. These terms can only serve to interfere with focus and erode concentration and confidence.

It is also essential to *encourage others*. The same awareness and consideration given to yourself should extend to your colleagues and team members because encouraging others yields positive benefits. Medical humor can often be macabre or sarcastic and used as a coping mechanism. However, excessive use, especially in the absence of encouragement and focus, can become a detrimental habit. Not only can it influence the reactions of others, but habitual sarcasm and negativism can make it more difficult to be encouraging to yourself.

The key to being able to STEP-UP is to *monitor and change self-talk* to promote performance. One way to do this is to use a STEP-UP Monitoring chart like this one:

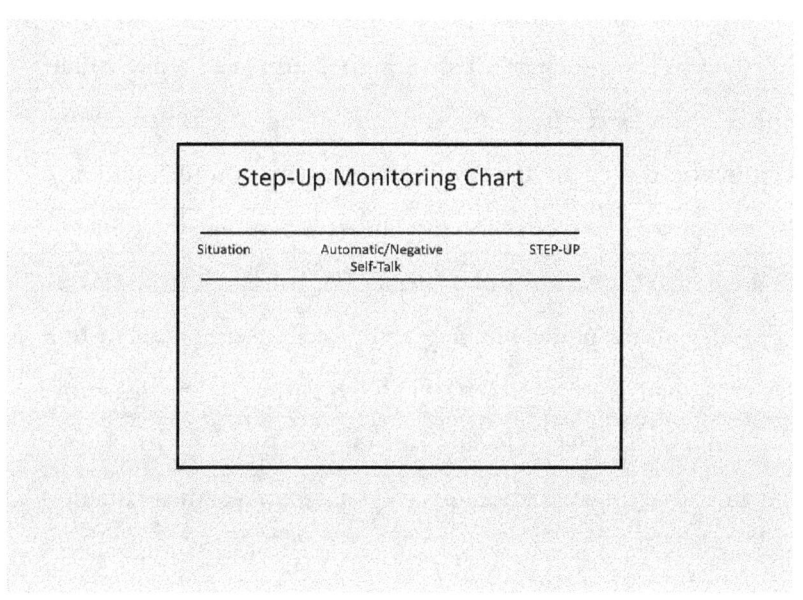

It is important to look for situations where you might engage in automatic non-productive and/or negative self-talk. Write the situation and the 'automatic' non-productive or negative self-talk in the first two columns. You might be able to do this by thinking about past situations where you became frustrated, upset, or stressed. Or, do it after a more recent encounter when memories and emotions are still fresh.

The crucial point is to then STEP-UP. Create and write in the third column alternate self-talk that will facilitate performance that is more effective.

The following chart illustrates an example of a potentially critical and stressful situation involving multiple trauma victims on top of an already busy shift with complex patients. By recognizing and charting the automatic or negative self-talk that creates distraction and dysfunction, you can become aware of irrelevant thoughts, any negativity and the source of further frustration. Also, note the STEP-UP response creates more functional and task relevant self-talk to be used to replace automatic or negative thoughts the next time a similar situation occurs.

Look at the STEP-UP column and see (feel) if these words do have a less upsetting effect and actually direct you to a more productive focus and action.

Step-Up Monitoring Chart

Situation	Automatic/Negative Self-Talk	STEP-UP
Multiple Trauma Victims In the Midst of an Already Busy Shift	I Can't Handle This Many Patients We Don't Have Enough Staff Tonight I'm Not Prepared for This What if People Die What if I Miss Something Important	Quick Triage ABC's and Repeat Call Trauma Surgery Activate Blood Bank ABC's Again

Now let's try your own STEPPING-UP. Use the chart below to write in your likely automatic (and probably negative) self-talk when encountering an unexpected cardiac arrest. Follow this by writing in what more effective self-talk or stepping-up might be. You can compare your responses to the ones suggested as examples in the next chart.

Step-Up Monitoring Chart

Situation	Automatic/Negative Self-Talk	STEP-UP
Unexpected Cardiac Arrest		

An example might be as below. We are not suggesting that this is the specific self-talk to use, but are giving an example; see if the automatic negative self-talk does, indeed, heighten arousal and anxiety while STEPPING-UP does suggest an action plan and better focus.

Self-talk in STEPPING-UP should be *focused on the behavior and action* you need to take to accomplish your goal. Murphy (1996) calls this an 'Action Focus' rather than a 'Results Focus.'

Step-Up Monitoring Chart

Situation	Automatic/Negative Self-Talk	STEP-UP
Unexpected Cardiac Arrest	I need help Isn't anyone here What if he dies!	Focus & Evaluate ABC's ACLS Algorithm

The Action focus in self-talk is more useful since it tells you how to get the result. If you perform the actions, the result should follow.

Your self-talk *should be brief.* Too much self-talk, or self-talk that is too involved or complicated, may be detrimental. Several studies (Mummert & Furley, 2007) now suggest that too much instruction can be a problem, especially for skilled performers, as it can interfere with well-learned and 'automatic' responses. Too much coaching and too much thinking lead to a narrowing of your attention, which may be a cause of decreased performance. This is an example of when 'analysis leads to paralysis.' It suggests that self-talk should be brief and direct.

A final approach to maximizing self-talk for enhanced performance is to *always phrase your self-talk positively in terms of what you should do, not what you should not do.* Telling yourself not to do something puts the focus exactly on what you want to avoid doing.

As an example, for the next two seconds, do not think of the ICU. What did you just think of? Most likely, an ICU! This is because of the six words in the statement telling you to not think of an ICU, the last four tell you to think about the ICU. Your mind has difficulty separating the 'do' from the 'do not' at the beginning of the sentence. A better STEP-UP for not thinking about the ICU would be 'think of the cafeteria.'

Wegner (1989) provides an anecdote that illustrates the impact of negative directives. It comes from Leo Tolstoy, author of the classic *War and Peace*, who as a child was ordered by his older brother to stand in a corner until he could stop thinking of a white bear! He goes on to note that the human brain isn't built to 'not think of something.' Phrasing it in the negative still puts the focus on what is to be ignored. Neurolinguistic

Programming offers that our brains 'simply do not know how to put things into negative language.' *In order to not think of something, you must first think of it* (Andreas & Faulkner, 1994).

This is an important concept since instructions are frequently phrased negatively in many types of training. How often in sports do you hear coaches say something like 'Don't strike out.' Where does that put the batter's focus? Or the classic advice when someone is in the situation of extreme heights (whether or not acrophobic) of 'Don't look down.'

Where does this focus the individual's attention and what does the individual do...usually immediately! Look down, of course. All of these types of instruction highlight the very actions that need to be avoided and do not offer a viable alternative. "Eyes on the ball" or "Eyes straight ahead" would be much more effective.

The same inadvertent misplaced focus can occur in nursing training and medical emergencies. Consider the admonition: *Don't contaminate the sterile field.* This, of course, focuses attention the very action to be avoided – contamination. Better phraseology might be: *Always exercise caution to maintain a sterile surgical field.*

Another example might be a diving accident or motor vehicle accident with a head injury.

An obvious instruction is often:

Don't move his neck.

Better phraseology might be:

Keep the neck in alignment.

or

Assure neck stabilization.

Even the classic medical dictum from Hippocrates of 'Primum no nocere' is a negative instruction:

First, do no harm.

Would it be better, if less eloquently phrased, as something like:

Always place patient safety, health and comfort first.

Nursing and medical training and texts actually do a rather good job of suggesting positive actions, rather than suggesting (even when cautioning) negative ones. It is important that we do the same in our personal thinking and self-talk. Becoming aware of and managing your self-talk can provide additional control for enhanced performance in high-stress situations.

Critical situations may not seem to allow time to 'think' or construct self-talk, especially since lengthy or complicated thinking can get in the way of executing skills effectively. While there is some truth to this, it does not negate the impact of self-talk on performance. It really argues for the importance of training and practice *prior* to critical situations, so that your self-talk is focused, direct, and powerful enough to promote appropriate action and excellence. It should be response-oriented.

Sometimes the need for Stepping-Up is not so much a crisis management technique as a means of need for self-control. There was the time a patient emptied her ostomy into the measuring container and threw it at me (KM) because she was mad at the doctor for not giving her more pain medication. What needed to be done to achieve a positive outcome was not to react negatively or impulsively. Although challenging, my performance-oriented self-talk in that immediate situation helped me keep a professional mindset in order to care for the patient for the rest of the shift. The incident occurred at the beginning of the shift. I was asked if I wanted to change patients or even press charges. I did not want to do either. I did not give her the opportunity to throw her stool contents at me again and I did manage to treat her, care for her needs and administer her medication, as well as, keeping a needed nurturant attitude to also attend to all my patients on that shift.

The practice and training of integrating mental and physical skills promotes their merging together into a more automatic and seamless response. By planning and practice, self-talk should become second nature, occurring automatically when needed. Whether you, indeed, **STEP-UP,** or whether your self-talk tears you down, depends on your mental preparation and practice.

IX. Mental Ablations: Negative Thought Stopping and Performance

To do what nobody else will do, in a way that nobody else can, in spite of all we go through; is to be a nurse.

-Rawsi Williams

There are many names for it: 'Toxic Thinking,' 'Stinkin' Thinkin',' 'Defeatist Attitude' and 'Negative Thinking.' Call it what you want, negative cognitive states can evolve from our self-talk and easily degrade performance. Understanding this process and, more importantly, developing effective interventions in addition to stepping-up to 'ablate' negative thinking is essential for maximizing your performance.

We said earlier that negative thinking or negative self-talk can interfere with optimal performance in emergency medical situations. It can do so by:

- Creating stress, anxiety, and depression
- Degrading self-confidence
- Distracting and reducing concentration
- Programming you for self-doubt
- Spreading to colleagues and team members
- Spreading to other areas of your life

Negativity erodes confidence and distracts you from the task at hand by putting your attention on an irrelevant, but disruptive focus. As a result, your concentration and creativity suffer. And the basis of cognitive control sees negative thoughts as instrumental in creating and maintaining anxiety and depression (Burns, 1981).

Negative thinking and negative self-talk affect your physiology, as well. Tennenbaum and his colleagues (2008) report research where subjects were exposed to a noxious traffic noise broadcast. Stress responses were evident in tachycardia and vasoconstriction. These effects were most pronounced in individuals who responded to the stressor with thoughts like "I can't handle this" or "This is making me crazy."

Negative thinking is at the root of self-doubt. The concept of a self-fulfilling prophecy says that our expectations about success or failure greatly influence our efforts and performance on a task. As Henry Ford said:

Whether you say "I can" or "I can't," you're right.

And paraphrasing the great president Thomas Jefferson:

Nothing can stop the person with the right mental attitude from achieving the goal; nothing on earth can help the person with wrong mental attitude.

It was discussed earlier that expectations exert powerful influences on our behavior. A study (or lore in sport psychology circles) was done on competitors at a national arm-wrestling championship (arm wrestling is apparently taken very seriously by some!). Each pair of finalists was tested for arm strength and each opponent was then given false feedback. The objectively stronger wrestler in the pair was told he was the weaker and the objectively weaker wrestler was told he was the stronger. In a majority of the final matches, the objectively weaker competitor, having been told he was stronger, won the event.

It is also important to note that negative expectations seem to be more influential than positive ones. That is, telling yourself that you will do something or that you will succeed may help motivation, but it does not guarantee success. *However, telling yourself that you cannot do something or that you cannot succeed will likely lead to failure and/or giving up.*

It takes a lot of effort to overcome the "toxicity of negative affect;" to fight back against performance degrading negative attitudes and feelings (Frederickson & Losada, 2006). What you need is a neutral problem-solving task-relevant focus for balance. The key, then, is to avoid negative thoughts and thinking (and also overly positive or unrealistic expectations). Positive expectations can help motivation, but even more effective is a problem-solving mode which, when combined with the correct task focus, can provide synergy to maximize performance, without interfering emotion and with direct suggestions for performance as in stepping-up..

Negative thinking is contagious; it easily spreads to others. You might have had the experience in which one person easily drags down a whole group. This is because negativity spreads more easily than does confidence. Maxwell (2001) calls this 'The Law of the Bad Apple.' We've all been around 'toxic' people who tend to bring out the worst in us. Every conversation centers on negative things and becomes a source of stress. It's best to limit contact with those individuals because that negativity can easily spread to other areas of your life and negative self-talk can become a destructive habit. And be sure you are not infectious to others because of your own negative thinking.

Elite military Special Forces members hate to hear someone whining or complaining. Interestingly though, this is not because they think the complaints are not valid, but rather because they believe whining means the person is not thinking about the right things to be successful; focus and concentration are off. If continuous whining is not addressed, it can hurt morale and ultimately lead to mission failure (Martin, 2006).

We are not suggesting that you always be positive and sunny. It would be unrealistic and artificial to be overly optimistic. However, we are suggesting that, in emergencies, you stay in an instructional, problem-solving mindset. Think about *what needs to be done to achieve a successful outcome*. Your self-talk should give you guidance as to how to act.

However, it's likely that even with the best attempts to stepping up and focus on stepping up, you will still have negative thoughts from time to time. Therefore, a technique called Negative Thought Stopping (NTS) can be helpful in managing your performance in high-stress situations. This is one of several techniques originally developed by Dr. Joseph Cautela at Boston University to help individuals gain greater control over negative thinking (1977). Although it's rather simple, it is easier to demonstrate than explain.

Here is how NTS is demonstrated in training. After discussing the toxic nature of negative thoughts, everyone is asked to close their eyes and think a negative or critical thought about themselves related to a recent stressful situation. After they have concentrated on the thought for about five seconds, the instructor suddenly slams his/her hand on the table or desk and yells as loudly as possible, 'Stop it!'

Everyone's eyes pop wide open as they sit bolt-upright and refocus their attention, trying to recover from their surprise.

The point being made with them, and confirmed when the participants are asked, is that the negative thought was completely ejected from their thinking and they are now focused back on the instructor. (It is always wise to check that everyone is heart-healthy before doing this demonstration!)

Here is the rationale and procedure for Negative Thought Stopping:

- Monitor for the presence of negative thoughts.
- If negative thoughts are present: Yell forcefully (internally) to yourself "NO" or "STOP IT"
- Give yourself a task-focused cue to refocus on the task.
- Continue to execute your skills.

As outlined above, whenever a negative thought enters your thinking, forcefully think (or 'yell' to yourself, not out loud!) the word 'No' or 'Stop it!' Then immediately give yourself a step-up cue like 'Focus,' 'Smooth,' 'Back to it,' or 'Treat' to focus on the skill you need to perform at that moment.

There are also several ways you can modify NTS. For some individuals, imaging a stop sign or a flashing neon sign that says 'NO' may be more effective than saying/thinking the word stop.

In another variation, you can add performance imagery to enhance your actions, cue your behavior, and help you refocus on the challenge. For example, after thinking "NO" or "STOP IT," immediately think of a task-focused cue, such as, 'CHECK VITALS,' and then image yourself scanning the monitor or checking a pulse. This will cue you to resume treatment where you left off. The use of reorienting commands like 'Check Vitals' or even just 'Focus' after NTS is essential for effectiveness.

NTS effectively returns your focus to positive actions. As with all psychological performance techniques, practice, and use enhance this skill.

Distraction not Suppression

Wegner (1989) has contributed much to our understanding of what makes the control of thinking effective. He notes that just trying to 'directly suppress' a thought is not effective. It is much like trying to, as he says, "not think of the color white." Remember, as discussed before, our minds are not designed to "not think of something."

In fact, trying directly to suppress a thought:

- Can cause you to focus on it even more
- Can cause a "rebound effect" where you think about the banished thought even more frequently after the suppression attempt is stopped
- Can, if you are not effective in suppressing the thought, cause an "intrusion reaction" in which the thought recurs, bringing with it a strong emotional response (usually negative)
- May cause a physiological response, usually a negative stress-type reaction

The use of distraction is much more effective. Distraction is thinking about something else, or replacing the unwanted thought with one or more others. Use a single thought or multiple thoughts as distracters (in fact, most people distract by using more than one thought). This works best when the thoughts are of great interest and significance to you.

Having considered, planned, developed, and practiced NTS and moderating distracting thoughts/self-statements prior to needing them makes their control at a critical moments much more likely.

X. Mental Clinical Pathways: Attitude, Affirmations & Performance

The character of a nurse is just as important as the knowledge he/she possesses

-Carolyn Jarvis

Selftalk and negative thought stopping intersect in the concept of attitude. They are the ingredients for creating and maintaining a successful attitude. This essential concept has been eloquently captured this way (Maxwell, 2002):

Attitude is the advance man of our true selves.
Its roots are inward, but its fruit outward.
It is our best friend and our worst enemy.
It is more honest and more consistent than our words.
It is an outward look based on past experiences.
It is a thing that draws people to us or repels them.
It is never content until it is expressed.

It is the librarian of our past.
It is the speaker of our present.
It is the prophet of our future.

Attitude is the essence of success and survival in stressful situations, whether acute or chronic. Hence, there is one other approach to maximizing attitude in addition to self-talk and NTS that is worth discussing briefly. This is the use of affirmations.

As mentioned earlier, you must be cautious when using positive thinking, encouragement, or affirmations because while there may be some effect on attitude, they do not provide direction and focus on *how* to maximize performance. However, with proper training and integration of the psychological skills discussed in this book, affirmations can contribute to the quality of performance by bolstering motivation and attitude. Perhaps the best source of successful attitude is your confidence in your ability to perform physically and psychologically, both of which can be enhanced by mastering mental performance skills.

Since, affirmations and their related positive thinking can affect your motivation, let's briefly examine them as they are commonly offered in other resources as a way to foster a productive mindset and a winning attitude.

Affirmations: What are They?

The nature and characteristics of affirmations are that:

- They are positive statements about ourselves that we make to ourselves.
- They are truthful statements as opposed to boasts which create unrealistic expectations or hopes.
- They remind us of our strengths, talents, skills, and goals.
- They work best when they are in the form of an "I" statement.
- They are most effective when stated in the present tense.
- They should be reviewed, stated, or meditated upon daily.

There are three typical categories of affirmations:

Personal Affirmations: These statements recognize your unique qualities.

I trust myself.

I am committed to excellence.

I always seek to improve myself.

I am confident in my ability to effectively care for my patients.

Professional Affirmations: These statements recognize your unique qualities as a nurse; they may also reflect the qualities of your team or service.

I am a dedicated nurse.

My team acts with professionalism, expertise, and integrity.

We take education and training seriously.

I make patient safety a priority.

Performance Affirmations: These statements recognize unique aspects of your skills and performance efforts.

In all duties and responsibilities, I take pride in my preparation.

I strive to maintain integrity in my actions at all times.

I always look out for my teammates.

I try to elevate the performance of all my team members.

What if you feel an affirmation is very important to you, but it is not yet true? If this is the case, it is more appropriately an 'aspiration' and it can be effective to change the wording to promote its potential (Andreas & Faulkner, 1994). For example you can replace "I am…:" with the phrasing "I can learn to be…" or "I will strive to develop…"

It is said that Ben Franklin wrote affirmations of his thirteen values and carried kept them in his pocket watch case. He had them with him at all times and frequently reviewed them whenever he checked the time (Andreas & Faulkner, 1994). Carry your pride with you.

Whether your path leads you to be an ordinary hero or an extraordinary hero in the eyes of a patient or your family, we hope the material in this book will help you summon your maximal skill in those moments of storm and challenge.

Appendix 1

CONCENTRATION GRID

23	12	07	15	62	93	82	36	21	37
31	50	59	28	46	30	25	48	69	76
45	49	73	19	02	67	04	77	41	64
26	29	88	03	34	13	91	38	56	86
87	83	98	35	43	44	24	39	40	20
90	96	89	80	42	94	53	05	55	57
61	75	65	32	22	11	08	10	27	09
00	99	95	85	14	01	74	60	92	31
18	51	71	54	63	17	79	33	70	52
97	78	58	84	06	16	66	72	47	68

References

Abramson, S., Stein, J., et al. (2000). Personal exercise habits and counseling practices of primary care physicians: A national survey. Clinical Journal of Sports Medicine, 10 (1),40- 8.

Abuissa, H., Lavie, C. et al. (2006). Personal health habits of American cardiologists. American Journal of Cardiology 97 (7), 1093-6.

Adams, S., Roxe, D., Weis, J., Zhang, F., & Rosenthal, J. (1998). Ambulatory blood pressure and holter monitoring of emergency physicians before, during and after a night shift. Academic Emergency Medicine, 5, (9), 871-877.

Afremow, James (2008). Personal communication. Health and Sport Psychology Clinic, Arizona State University.

Alexander, J., Groller, R., & Morris, J. (1990). The Warrior's Edge. NY: William Morrow.

Alger S, Berger A, & Capaldi V. Challenging the stigma of workplace napping. Sleep, 2019: 48 (8), 1-2 zsz097 https://doi.org/10.1093/sleep/zsz097

Andreas, S., & Faulkner, C. (1994). NLP: The New Technology of Achievement. New York: Harper

Anton, N., Beane, J., Yurco, A., Howley, L., Bean, E., Myers, E., & Stefanidis, D. (2018). Mental skills training effectively minimize operative performance deterioration under stressful conditions: Results of a randomized controlled study. American Journal of Surgery. 215:214-221.

Anton, N., Mizota, T., Whiteside, J., Myers, M., Bean, E., & Stefanidis, D. (2019). Mental skills training limits the decay of operative technical skill under stressful conditions: Results of a multisite, randomized controlled study. American Journal of Surgery.165: 1059-1064.

Anton, N., Bean, E., Hammonds, S., & Stefanidis, D. (2017). Application of mental skills training in surgery: A review of its effectiveness and proposed next steps. Journal of Laparoendoscopic & Advanced Surgical Techniques. 27:459-469.

Anton, N., Zhou, G., Hornbek, T., Nagle, A., Norman, S., Shroff, A., & Yu, D. (2023). Detailing experienced nurse decision-making during acute patient care simulations. Applied Ergonomics. 109:103988

Arora, S., Aggarwal, R., Sirimanna, P., Moran, A., Grantcharov, T., Kneebone, R., Darzi, A. (2011). Mental practice enhances surgical technical skills: A randomized controlled study. Annals of Surgery, 253 (2): 265-270.

Artwohl, A. (2002) Perceptual and memory distortion during officer involved shootings. FBI Law Enforcement Bulletin. 2002; October, 71 (10): 18-24.

Artwohl, A, & Christensen, L. (1997) Deadly Force Encounters. 1997; Boulder Co: Paladin Press

Asken M. (2020). Code Calm: Mental Toughness Skills for Optimal Response in Medical Emergencies. Amazon E-books.

Asken M, Owens, R, & Ladie D. (2023). MindBenders: Stress as a perception distorting prism in surgery. General Surgery News: January
https://www.generalsurgerynews.com/Opinion/Article/01-23/Intraoperative-Stress/69143

Asken, M. Zuniga, P. & Safaee, S. (2001). Code Cool: Psychological skills training to reduce anticipatory anxiety in medical residents in code situations. Medical Education Day, Pinnacle Health System, Harrisburg, PA., March.

Asken, M. (1993). PsycheResponse: Psychological Skills for Optimal Response by Emergency Responders. Englewood Cliffs, NJ: Brady-Prentice Hall.

Asken, M. (2005). MindSighting: Mental Toughness Training for Police Officers in High Stress Situations. Camp Hill, PA.

Asken, M., Yang, H., Aboushi, R., & Paulovich, K. (2020). Prepping for Surgery: Surgeon Prepare Thyself. American Journal of Surgery. 21 (4): 75-76.

Asken, M & Jensen, N. (2021) What sports training can teach medical education. Meedical Economics. November 30. https://www.medicaleconomics.com/view/what-sports-training-can-teach-medical-education-one-lesson-worth-considering

Asken, M., & Yang, H. (2021). SIM: The Surgeon's Imagery MindSet. Amazon e-Books.

Asken, M., Shrimanker, I., Bhattari, S. Nookala, V., & Slaven, V, (2020). Code Calm: BLS/ACLS training, mindset training, anticipatory anxiety and confidence in interns. Submitted for publication.

Atkinson JW. *An introduction to motivation.* 1964; Princeton, N. J: D. Van Nostrand

Bachman, K. (1990). Using mental imagery to practice a specific psychomotor skill. Journal of continuing education in Nursing. 21 (3), 125-128.

Bakhamis L, Paul D, Smith H, et al. Still an epidemic: The burnout syndrome in hospital registered nurses. The Health Care Manager. 2019; 38 (1): 3-10.

Barnard, J., Macalpin, R., Kattus, A., & Buckberg, G. (1973). Ischemic response to sudden strenuous exercise in healthy men. Circulation, 48, 936-942.

Bathalon, S., Dorion, D., Darveau, S., & Martin, M. (2005). Cognitive skills analysis, kinesiology, and mental imagery in the acquisition of surgical skills. Otolaryngology, 34, (5), 328-32.

Baubin, M., Schirmer, M., Nogler, M., et al. (1996). Rescuer's work capacity and duration of cardiopulmonary resuscitation. Resuscitation, 33, (2), 135-139.

Barrett, M. (2006). Cited in Repetition reverses med students' stethoscope shortcomings. Science Daily. January 18, www.sciencedaily.com.

Behavioral Physiology Institute (2008). CapnoLearningTM. Boulder, CO: www.bp.edu. Beilock S. Choke: What the secrets of the brain reveal about getting it right when you have to. New York: Free Press, 2010.

Begley, S. (2007). What the Beatles gave science. Newsweek, November, 19, p.59.

Benson, H. (1975). The Relaxation Response. NewYork: Morrow.

Bertram, C. (2023). Flow. The Emergency Mind Podcast. March. www.emergencymind.com/podcast

Blake, H., Malik, S., Phoenix, K., Pisano, C. (2011). 'Do s I say, but not do as I do: 'Are next generation nurses role models for health? Perspective in Public Health. 131 (5), 231-239.

Boehm, l. & Tse, A. (2013). Application of guided imagery to facilitate the transition of new graduate nurses. Journal of Continuing Education in Nursing. 44 (3), 113-119.

Bohm, B., Rotting, N., Schwenk, W., Grebe, S., & Mansmann, U. (2001). A prospective randomized trial on heart rate variability of the surgical team during laparoscopic and conventional sigmoid resection. Archives of Surgery, 136, 305-309.

Bond, W., Kuhn, G., Binstadt, E., et al. (2008). The use of simulation in the development of individual cognitive expertise in emergency medicine. Academic Emergency Medicine, 15, 1037-1045.

Bucher, K. (1993). The effects of imagery abilities and mental rehearsal on learning a nursing skill. Journal of Nursing Education. 32 (7), 318-324.

Burns, D. (1981). Feeling Good: The New Mood Therapy. New York: William Morrow.

Capelle, C., & Paul, R. (1996). Educating residents: The effect of a mock code program. Resuscitation, 3, 107-111.

Carey, C. (2004). The neurobiology of the placebo effect: A review. http://staff.washington.edu/ccarey/placebo

Causer, J., Vickers, J., Snelgrove, R., Arsenault, G., & Harvey, J. (2014). Surgery. 156 (5):1089-1096.

Cautela J., & Wisocki, P. (1977). The thought-stopping procedure: Description, application and learning theory interpretations. The Psychological Record. 27: 255-264.

Christensen, L. (1999). The Mental Edge Revised. El Dorado, AZ: Desert Publications.

Clark, L. (1960). Effects of mental practice on the development of a certain motor skill. Research Quarterly, 31, 560-569.

Contrades, S. (1991). Guided imagery use in nursing education. Journal of Holistic Nursing. June,
https://doi.org/10.1177/089801019100900206

Cooper, G. (2008). Hospital Survival: Lessons Learned in medical Training. Philadelphia: Lippincott/Williams & Wilkins

Cromie, W. (2002). Meditation changes temperatures: Mind controls body in extreme experiments. Harvard University Gazette, April 18, www.hno.harvard.edu/gazette/2002/04.18/09-tummo.html

Csikszentmihalyi, M. (1990). Flow: The Psychology of Optimal Experience. New York: Harper.

Cuddy, A. (2015) Presence: Bringing Your Boldest Self to Your Biggest Challenges. New York: Little Brown & Company.

Cuddy, A. (2016). More confidence in two minutes. https://www.youtube.com/watch?v=r7dWsJ-mEyI&t=2s

Cumming, J., Olphin, T., et al., (2007). Self-reported psychological states and physiological responses to different types of motivational general imagery. Journal of Sport and Exercise Psychology, 29, 629-644.

Descahumes-Molinaro, C., Dittmar, A., & Vernet-Maury, E. (1992). Autonomic nervous system response patterns correlate with mental imagery. Physiological Behavior, 51 (5), 1021-1027

Dingfelder, S. (2007). Your brain on video games. Monitor on Psychology, 38, (2), 20-21.

Di Nasio, J. (2006). The Law of Exercise Specificity: Is your workout real to help you in the field? www.policeone.com, 06-05-2006.

Dishman R. Exercise compliance: A new perspective in public health. The Physician and SportsMedicine. 1986: 14(5):127-145.

Doheny, M. (1993). Effects of mental practice on performance on a psychomotor skill. Journal of Mental Imagery.17 (3-4), 111-118.

Driskell, J., Salas, E., & Johnston, J. (2006). Decision making and performance under stress. In T. Britt, C. Castro, & A. Adler (Eds.). Military Life: The Psychology of Serving in Peace and Combat. Volume I: Military Performance, 128-154.

Drummond, D., Delval, P., Abdenouri, S. et al. (2017). Serious game versus online course pre-training medical students before simulation-based mastery learning course on cardiopulmonary resuscitation. European Journal of Anaesthesiology, 34: 836-844.

Duran, P. (1999). Developing the Survival Attitude. NY: Looseleaf.

Eaton, S., & Evans, S. (1986). The effect of non-specific imaging practice on the mental imagery ability of nursing students. Journal of nursing education. 25 (5), 193-196.

Eichner R. Overtraining: Consequences and prevention. Journal of Sport Sciences. 1995: 13, Supp 1, S41-S48.

Elkins, G. (2016). Handbook of Medical and Psychological Hypnosis. Berlin: Springer.

Ericsson, K. (2008). Deliberate practice and acquisition of expert performance: A general overview. Academic Emergency Medicine, 15, 988-994.

Feltovich, P., Prietula, M., & Ericsson, K. (2006). Studies of expertise from psychological perspectives. In K. Ericsson, N. Charness, P. Feltovich, &. R. Hoffman, (Eds.). The Cambridge Handbook of Expertise and Expert Performance. Cambridge, England: Cambridge University Press.

Fernandez, R., Vozenilik, J., Hegarty, C. et al., (2008). Developing expert medical teams: Toward an evidenced-based approach. Academic Emergency Medicine, 15, 1025-1036.

Ferrell, M., Beach, R., Szeverneyi, N. (2006). An fMRI analysis of neural activity during perceived zone-state performance. Journal of Sport and Exercise Psychology, 28, 421-433.

Flin, R., Youngson, G., & Yule, S. (2016). Enhancing Surgical Performance: A Primer in non-technical skills. Boca Raton: CRC Press.

Fountaki, A., Kotrotsiou, S., Paralikas T., Malliarou, M., Konstanti, Z., Tsioumanis G., & Theofanidis, D. (2021). Professional mental rehearsal: The power of "imagination" in nursing skills training. Mater Sociomed: 33 (3):174-178.

Frederickson, B., & Losada, M. (2006). Positive affect and the complex dynamics of human flourishing. *American Psychologist*. 60 (7), 678-686.

Frank, E., Bhat-Schelbert, K. et al., (2003). Exerxcise counseling and personal exercise hanbits of US women physicians. Journal of the American Medical Women's Association, 58 (3), 178-184

Gauron, E. (1984). Mental Training for Peak Performance. Lansing, NY: Sport Science Assoc.

Gawande,A. (2007). Better: A Surgeon's Notes on Performance. NY: Picador

Ghannam, C. (2009). Military, police trainer and performance enhancement innovator. Personal Communication. www.sarksecurities.com.

Geiger-Brown J, Sagherian K, Zhu S, et al. Napping on night shift: A two hospital implementation project. AJN: 2016: 16 (5), 26-33.https://nursing.ceconnection.com/ovidfiles/00000446-201605000-00027.pdf

Gibson, L. (2006). Nightmares: A National Center for PTSD fact sheet. www.ncptsd.va.gov.

Goldberg, R., Boss, R., Goldberg, J., Mallon, W., et al., (1996). Burnout and its correlates in emergency physicians: Four years' experience with a wellness booth. Academic Emergency Medicine, 3, (12), 1156-1164.

Goodspeed, R. & Lee, B. (2007). What If…?: A survival Guide for Physicians. Philadelphia: F.A. Davis.

Graham, D. (n.d.) Where did Hemingway say courage is grace under pressure? https://www.quora.com/Where-did-Hemingway-say-courage-is-grace-under-pressure

Graham, G. (2010). Operational risk management. South Central Emergency Task Force Health and Safety Conference. Harrisburg Area Community College, Harrisburg, PA: 02-06-2010.

Grant, C. (Eds.). Success strategies for women in STEM. 2015: NY: Academic Press.

Green, S., & Bavelier, D. (2006). Effect of action video games on the spatial distribution of visual attention. Journal of Experimental Psychology: Human perception and performance, 32,(6), 1465-1478.

Griffin, M, & Cooper, C. (2006). Using near-infrared spectroscopy to "measure" imagery. NASPSPA Abstracts 2006, Journal of Sport and Exercise Psychology, 28, 576-577.

Grossman, D., & Christensen, L. (2008). On Combat. Warrior Science Press: Milstadt, IL.

Guillot, A. Collet, C., Molinaro, CV. & Dittmar, A. (2004). Expertise and peripheral autonomic activity during the preparation phase in shooting events. *Perceptual and Motor Skills*, 98 (2), 371-381.

Hall, J. (2002). Imagery practice and the development of surgical skills. The American Journal of Surgery, 184. 465-470.

Hancock, P. (2009). Performance on the very edge. Military Psychology, 21 (Suppl. I), S68-S64.

Hancock, P., & Szalma, J. (2008). Stress and performance. In P. Hancock & J. Szalma (Eds.). Performance Under Stress. Hampshire, England: Ashgate Publishing Limited.

Hansen, A., Johnsen, B., & Thayer, J. (2008). Relationship between heart rate variability and cognitive function during threat of shock. Anxiety, Stress & Coping, 9, 1-12.

Hart, P., Brannan, J., De Chesnay, M. (2014). Resilience in nurses: An integrative review. Journal of Nursing Management. 22 (6),720-734.

Harvey, A., Vickers, J., Snelgrove, R., Scott, M., & Morrison, S. (2014). The American Journal of Surgery. 207 (2):187-193.

Hawkins, J. (2004). On Intelligence. New York: Henry Holt and Company

Helin, P., Sihvonen, T., & Hanninen, O. (1987). Timing of the triggering action of shooting in relation to the cardiac Cycle. British Journal of Sports Medicine, 21 (1), 33-36.

Hendricks, M. (2000). Physician, writer, philosopher, sage. Johns Hopkins Magazine, 52, (2), 65.

Hicks, C., Bandiera, G., Denny, C., et al. (2008). Building a simulation-based crisis resource management course for emergency medicine Phase 1: Results from an interdisciplinary needs assessment survey. Academic Emergency Medicine, 15, 1136-1143.

Hill, N., and Schneider, W. (2006). Brain changes in the development of expertise: Neuroanatomical and neurophysiological evidence about skill-based adaptations. In K. Ericsson, N. Charness, P. Feltovich, &. R. Hoffman, (Eds.). The Cambridge Handbook of Expertise and Expert Performance. Cambridge, England: Cambridge University Press.

Hinkle, J., Cheever, K., & Overbaugh, K. (2022). Brunner and Suddharth's Textbook of Medical Surgical Nursing. Philadelphia: Wolters Kluwer.

Holmes, P. & Collins, D. (2001). The PETTLEP approach to motor imagery: A functional equivalence model for sport psychologists. Journal of Applied Sport Psychology. 13:60-83.

Holmstedt, K. (2007). Band of Sisters: American Women at War in Iraq. Mechanicsburg, PA: Stackpole Books.

Honig, A., & Sultan, S. (2004). Reactions and resilience under fire. What an officer can expect. The Police Chief, 71, (12), www.policechief.org.

Houry, D., Shockley, L., & Markovchick, V. (2000). Wellness issues and the emergency medicine resident. Annals of Emergency Medicine, 35,(4), 394-397.

Hunziker S., Pagani, S., Fasier K., Tschan F., Semmer N., & Marsch, S. (2013). Impact of a stress coping strategy on perceived stress levels and performance during a simulated cardiopulmonary resuscitation: a randomized controlled trial. BMC Emergency Medicine. 13:8.

Ignacio, J., Dolmans D., Scherpbier, A., Rethans, J., Lopez V., & Liaw S. (2016). Development, implementation and evaluation of a mental rehearsal strategy to improve clinical performance and reduce stress: A mixed methods study. Nursing Education Today. (37): 32.

Ignacio, J., Scherpbier, A., Dolmans, D., Rethans J., Liaw, S. (2017). Mental rehearsal strategy for stress management and performance in simulations. Clinical Simulation in Nursing. 13 (7): 295-302.

Immenroth, M., Burger, T., Brenner, J., et al. (2007). Mental training in surgical education: A randomized controlled trial. Annals of Surgery, 245, (3), 385-391.

Institute of Medicine (2007). Hospital-Based Emergency Care: At the Breaking Point. Washington, DC: national Academy of Sciences, National Academies Press.

Jadick, R. (2007). On Call in Hell: A Doctor's Iraq War Story. New York, NAL Caliber.

Jain, A., Thompson, J., Chaudry, J., et al., (2008). High performance teams for current and future physician leaders. Journal of Surgical Education. www.sciencedirect.com, 11-14-2008.

Janelle, C., & Hatfield, B. (2008). Visual attention and brain processes that underlie expert performance: Implications for sport and military psychology. Military Psychology, 20 (Suppl. 1), S39-S69.

Janelle, C., Hillman, C. et al. (2000) Expertise differences in cortical activation and gaze Behavior during rifle shooting. Journal of Sport & Exercise Psychology, 22(2) 167-182

Janis, I. (1973). Victims of Groupthink: A Psychological Study of Foreign Policy Decisions and Fiascos. Boston: Houghton-Mifflin.

Jensen N & Asken, M. (2021). What sports training can teach medical education. Medical Economics. November 30. https://www.medicaleconomics.com/view/what-sports-training-can-teach-medical-education-one-lesson-worth-considering

Jinks, A. & Daniels, R. (2003). A survey of the health needs of hospital staff: Implications for health care managers. Journal of Nursing Management. 11, 343-352.

Johnson, A., Jung, L., Brown, K. (2014). Sleep deprivation and error in nurses who work night shift. The Journal of Nursing Administration. 44 (1), 17-22.

Kabat-Zinn, J. (2016). Mindfulness for beginners. Boulder, Colorado: Sounds True Publishing.

Kaewthummanukul, T., Brown, K., Weaver, M., & Thomas, R. (2006). Predictors of exercise participation in female hospital nurses. Journal of Clinical Nursing. 54 (6), 663-675.

Kahneman, D. (2013).Thinking, Fast and Slow. NY: Farrar, Straus& Giroux.

Kay, J. (2007). Army medical units tackle trauma under pressure. The Sunday Patriot News, 10-28-2007, A20.

Kavanagh, J. (2005). Stress and Performance: A Review of the Literature and Its Applicability to the Military. Santa Monica, CA: Rand Corporation.

Klein, G. (2003). The Power of Intuition. New York: Currency.

Koltnow, S. (2004). Physician well-being. In J. Tintanalli, G. Kalen, & J. Stapczynski. Emergency Medicine: A Comprehensive Study Guide. NY: McGraw-Hill.

Krage, R., Len, T., Schober,P., et al. (2014). Does individual experience affect performance during cardioplulmonary resuscitation with additional external distractors. Anaesthesia. 19 (9), 983-989.

Krakow, B., et al. (2001). Imagery rehearsal therapy for chronic nightmares in sexual assault survivors with post-traumatic stress disorder: A randomized controlled trial. Journal of the American Medical Association, 286 (5), 537-545.

Krischke, M. (2013). RN warning: Irregular sleep can be dangerous. Nursing Education.
https://www.rn.com/nursing-news/warning-irregular-sleep-can-be-dangerous/

Lammers,R., Davenport, M., Korley, F., et al., (2008). Teaching and assessing procedural skills using simulation: Metrics and Methodology. Academic Emergency Medicine, 15, 1079-1087.

Lauria, M., Gallo, I., Rush, S., Brooks, J. Spiegel, R., & Weingart, S. (2017). Psychological skills to improve emergency care providers' performance under stress. Ann Emerg Med. 70:884-890.

Laws, T. (2001). Examining critical care nurses' critical incident stress after in hospital cardiopulmonary resuscitation (CPR). Australian Critical Care, 14 (2), 76-81.

LeBlanc. V., & Bandiera, G. (2007). The effects of examination stress on the performance of emergency medicine residents. Medical Education, 41, (6), 556-564.

Levitan, R. Butler, K., & Asken, M. 2015. Unpublished data.

Lichtenstein, K. (1988). Clinical Relaxation Strategies. New York: John Wiley.

Lieberman, H., Bathalon, G., et al., (2005). The fog of war: Decrements in cognitive performance and mood associated with combat-like stress. Aviation, Space Environmental Med, Jul, 76 (7 suppl) C7-14.

Lima, E., Knopfholz, J., & Menini, C. (2002). Stress during ACLS courses: is it important for learning skills? Arq Bras Cardiology, 79, (6), 589-592.

Lippincott Solutions (2017). Predicting postcode PTSD. Lippincottsolutions.lww.com/blog.entry.html/2017/03/23/predicting_postcode-IVhg.html

Magtibay D., Chesal, S., Coughlin, K., et al. (2017). Decreasing stress and burnout in Nurses. The Journal of Nursing Administration. 47 (7/8), 391-395.

Makinen, M., Neimi-Murola, L., Kaila, M., et al. (2009). Nurses' attitudes towards resuscitation and national resuscitation guidelines-Nurses hesitate to start CPR-D. Resuscitation, 80 (12), 1399-1404.

Martin K. Combating mental fatigue in soldiers. J Sci Med Sport. 2017:(20): S53-S54.

May, J., & Asken, M., (1987). Sport Psychology: The Psychological Health of the Athlete. NY:PMA Publishing.

Maxwell, J. (2001). The 17 Indisputable Laws of Teamwork. Nashville: Thomas Nelson.

Martin, J. (2006). Get Selected for Special Forces. Yuma, AZ: Warrior-Mentor Press.

Maurer, H., & Munzert, J. (2005). Can "choking under pressure" be explained by an internal focus of attention? A study with expert basketball players. NASPSPA Abstracts, Journal of Sport & Exercise Psychology, S14.

McCann, K. (2010). Lapses of attention and reaction time in sleep-deprived nurses working successive 12-hour shifts. San Antonio: Sleep Conference June.

McClelland D. Human Motivation. 1988. Cambridge, UK: Cambridge University Press.

McNamara, R., & Margulies, J. (1994). Chemical dependency in emergency medicine residency programs: perspective of the directors. Annals of Emergency Medicine, 23, (5),1072-1076.

Mealer, M., Conrad, D., Evans, J., et al. (2014). Feasibility and acceptability of a resilience training program for intensive care unit nurses. American Journal of Critical Care. 23 (6), e97-105.

Mealer, M., Hodapp, R., Conrad, D., et al. (2017). Designing a resilience program for critical care nurses. AACN Advanced Critical Care. 28 (4), 359-365.

Meekin, D., Hickman, R., Douglas, S. et al. (2017). Stress and coping of critical nurses after unsuccessful cardiopulmonary resuscitation. American Journal of Critical Care 26 (2), 128-135.

Meichenbaum, D. (1985). Stress Inoculation Training. Elmsford, NY: Pergamon Press.

Metcalfe, J. (2014). FDNY Optimal performance seminar. Palisades, NY.

Miller, L. (2007). Mettle: Mental toughness training for law enforcement. Flushing, NY: Looseleaf Law Publications.

Mills, K. (2005). Disciplined Attention: How To Improve Your Visual Attention When You Drive. Chapel Hill, NC: Profile Press.

Mindful Staff (2017). Jon Kabat-Zinn: Defining mindfulness. https://www.mindful.org/jon-kabat-zinn-defining-mindfulness/

Moran, A. (1996). The Psychology of Concentration in Sport Performers: A Cognitive Analysis. East Sussex, UK: Psychology Pres, Taylor & Francis.

Morris, T., Spittle, M., & Watt, A. (2005). Imagery In Sport. Champaign, Ill: Human Kinetics. Mullins, W. (2003). The effects of caffeine and caffeine withdrawal/deprivation on hostage negotiator performance. Journal of Police Crisis Negotiations, 3, (2), 39- 60.

Moseley, J., O'Malley, K., Petersen, N., et al (2002). A controlled trial of arthroscopic knee surgery for osteoarthritis of the knee. New England Journal of Medicine, 347 (2), 81-88.

Moss, D., Lehrer, P., & Gevirtz, R. (2008). Special issue: The emergent science and practice of heart rate variability biofeedback. Biofeedback, 36, (10), 1-4.

Mummert, D., & Furley, P. (2007). "I spy with my little eye": Breadth of attention, inattentional blindness and tactical decision making in team sports. Journal of Sport and Exercise Psychology, 29, 365-381.

Murphy, S. (1996). The Achievement Zone. New York: Putnam.

Murphy, S. (2005). Imagery: Inner theater becomes reality. In S. Murphy (ed.) The Sport Psych Handbook. Champaign, Il: Human Kinetics.

Murray, K. Training at the Speed of Life. (2004). Gotha, Fl: Armiger Publications.

Naintas D. LSU showcases insane new football facility after 28 million dollar renovation. Sporting News, July 2019.

Nideffer, R. (1985). Athlete's Guide to Mental Training. Champaign, Il: Human Kinetics.

Nideffer, R., & Sharpe, R. (1978). Attention Control Training: How to Get Control of Your Mind Through Total Concentration. New York: WideView Books.

Nowicki, D. (1994). Gold Medal Mental Workout for Combat Sports. Island Pond, VT: Stadion.

Nurenberg, E. & Asken, M. (2014) FirePsyche: Mental Toughness and the VALOR Mindset for the Fireground. New York: Leadership Under Fire.

Ochoa, F., Ramalle-Gomara, E., Lisa, V., et al. (1998). The effect of rescuer fatigue on the quality of chest compressions. Resuscitation, 37, (3), 149-152.

Pargman, D. (2006). Managing Performance Stress. London: Brunner-Routledge.

Peng, X. & Dongmei, W. 2022. The protective effect of grit on clinical nurses' occupational psychological distress: Mediating and suppressing effects of Hope. Frontiers in Psychology: Published online 2022 Sep 29. doi: 10.3389/fpsyg.2022.1019655

Perry, C. (2005). Concentration: Focus under pressure. In S. Murphy (Ed.). Sport Psych Handbook. Champaign, Il: Human Kinetics.

Perry, A., Potter P., & Ostendorf, W. Clinical Nursing Skills and Techniques. 9th Edition. St. Louis: Elsevier.

Peynircioglu, Z. (2000). Improvement strategies in free-throw shooting and grip-strength tasks. Journal of General Psychology, (Apr). www.findarticles.com.

Potter, P., Perry, A. Stockert, P. et al. Fundamentals of Nursing. 11th Ed. 2023. St. Louis: Elsevier.

Price, M. (2008). Testing makes perfect, finds memory retrieval research. APAMonitor on Psychology, 39, (6), 11. Pritchard, P. & Grant, C. (Eds.). Success strategies for women in STEM. 2015: NY: Academic Press.

PT Direct. Attendance, Adherence Retention and Drop Out. 2023:https://www.ptdirect.com/training-design/exercise-behaviour-and-adherence/attendance-adherence-drop-out-and-retention-patterns-of-gym-members

Rahman, M. (2007). A Discourse on Law Enforcement and Psychobehaviors: Informing Design Displays from Displays in Ethology to High Velocity Human Factors (Tech Report DHF-KFM-1) Plantation, Fl: Design International, Motorola. (Copies may be obtained from the author at: moin.rahman@motorola.com.)

Purvis, D, Gonsalves, S, Deuster, P. Physiological and Psychological Fatigue in Extreme Conditions: The Elite Athlete. PM&R. 2010:2(5): 442-450.

Ranse, J. (2008). Graduate nurses' lived experience of in-hospital resuscitation: a hermeneutic phenomenological approach. Australian Critical Care, 21, (1), 38-47.

Raso, R. (2021). Mental toughness – When it isn't enough. Nursing Management. October:4.

Remsberg, C. (1986). The Tactical Edge. Northbrook, Il: Calibre Press.

Richardson, A. (1969). Mental Imagery. London: Routledge & Keegan Paul.

Richardson, M. (2011). Developing mental toughness. Mental Health Nurses Leadership Academy. Nursing Times. https://www.nursingtimes.net/roles/mental-health-nurses/developing-mental-toughness

Salas, E., DiazGranados, D., Weaver, S., et al., (2008), Does team training work? Principles for health care. Academic Emergency Medicine, 15, 1002-1009.

Sanders, C., Sadoski, M., van Walsum, K, et al., (2008). Learning basic surgical skills with mental imagery: Using the simulation centre in the mind. Medical Eucation, 42, (6), 607-612.

Santos, A. (2016). Nurse's guide to mental imagery. Nursing 2020. 46 (1), 55-58. Scarborough J. Roman medicine and the legions: A reconsideration. Med History. 1968:12 (3), 254-261.

Schaider, J., Hayden, S., Wolfe, R., Barkin, R., Rosen, P. (2007, 3rd Ed). Rosen and Barkin's 5 Minute Emergency Medicine Consult. Philadelphia: Lippincott, Williams & Wilkins.

Schultz, J. H., & Luthe, W. (1959). *Autogenic training: A psychophysiologic approach to psychotherapy.* New York: Grune & Stratton.

Schwartz, M. & Andrasik, F. (2017) Biofeedback: A practitioner's guide. New York: Guilford Press.

Semeraro, F., Signore, L., & Cerchiari, E., (2005). Retention of CPR performance in anaesthetists. Resuscitation, Nov.

Siddle. B. (2009). The stress paradox. The War on Trauma: Lessons Learned From a Decade of Conflict. Supplement to the Journal of Emergency Medical Services, October, 2008, 28-31.

Skorski S, Mujika I, Bosquet L, Meeusen R, Coutts A, Meyer T. The temporal relationship between exercise, recovery processes and changes in performance. International Journal of Sports Physiology and Performance. 2019: 14, 1015-1021

Small, S. (2007). Simulation applications for human factors and systems evaluation. Anesthesiology Clinics, 25, (2), www.mdconsult.com, 10-15-2008.

Smith, D. (2006). Psychology and body building. In J. Dosil (Ed.). The Sport Psychologist's Handbook: A Guide for Sport-Specific Performance Enhancement. New York: John Wiley, 618-639.

Sok, S., Kim, J., Lee, Y. et al. (2020) Effects of a simulation-based CPR training program on knowledge, performance and stress in clinical knowledge. The Journal of continuing Education in nursing, 51 (5), 225-232.

Sonnon, S. (2001). Keeping the Edge: Flow State Performance Spiral. Atlanta, GA: AARMACS.

Soohoo, S., Takemoto, K., & McCullagh, P. (2004). A comparison of modeling and imagery on the performance of a motor skill. Journal of Sport Behavior, 27, (4), 349-366.

Spierer D., Griffiths E., Sterling T. (2009). Fight or flight: Measuring and understanding human stress response in tactical situations. The Tactical Edge. 2009, Summer, 30-40

Staal, M., Bolton, A., Yarowish, R. et al., (2008). Cognitive performance and resilience to stress. In Lukey, B., & Tepe, V. (eds.) Biobehavioral Resilience to Stress. Boca Raton, FL: CRC Press.

Starr, L. (1987). Stress inoculation training applied to cardiopulmonary resuscitation. Paper presented at the 95th Annual Meeting of the American Psychological Association, New York, New York.

Stefanidis, D., Anton, A., Howley, L., Bean, E., Yurco, A., Pimental, M., & Davis, C. (2017). Effectiveness of a comprehensive mental skills curriculum in enhancing surgical performance: Results of a randomized controlled trial. American Journal of Surgery. 13: 318-324.

St. Pierre, M., Hofinger, G, Buerchaper, C., & Simon, R. (2011). Crisis Management in Acute Care Settings. Berlin: Springer-Verlag.

Stephens, R. (1992). Imagery: a treatment for nursing student anxiety. Journal of Nursing Education. 31(7), 314-320.

Strentz, T. (2006). Psychological Aspects of Crisis Negotiation. Boca Raton, FL: CRC.

Suinn, R. (1980). Psychology and sport performance: Principles and applications. In R. Suinn (Ed.). Psychology in Sports: Methods and Applications. Minneapolis, Mn: Burgess.

Suinn, R. (1985) Imagery rehearsal applications to performance enhancement. *The Behavior Therapist,* 8 (9), 179-183.

Tennenbaum, G., Edmonds, W., & Eccles, D. (2008). Emotions, coping strategies, and performance: A conceptual framework for defining affect-related performance zones. Military Psychology, 20, (Suppl. 1), S11-S37.

Terry, D. & Peck, B. (2020). Academic and clinical performance among nursing students: What's grit got to do with it. Nurse EducationToday88:https://www.sciencedirect.com/science/article/abs/pii/S0260691719313255

Thompson, M., & McCreary, D. (2006). Enhancing mental readiness in military personnel. In T. Britt, C. Castro, & A. Adler (Eds.). Military Life: The Psychology of Serving in Peace and Combat, Volume 1: Military Performance, New York: Praeger, 54-79.

Torquati, L., Pavey, T. Kolbe-Alexander, T., Leveritt, M. (2017). Promoting diet and physical activity in nurses: A systematic review. American Journal of Health Promotion. 31 (1) 19-27.

Tosunoz I., Oztunc G. Low back pain in nurses. International Journal of Caring Sciences. 2017; 10 (3):1728.

Urden, S., Stacy, K., & Lough, M. (2018). Critical Care Nursing. Maryland Heights, Mo: Elsevier.

Van Tilburg, C. (2007). Mountain Rescue Doctor. New York: St. Martin's Press.

Vickers, J. (2016) Origina and issue sin Quiet Eye Research. Current Issues in Sports Science. 1, 1-11. https://www.momentum-quarterly.org/ojs2/index.php/ciss/article/view/36/4

Vranich, B. (2016). Breathe. New York: St. Martin's Press.

Wang, E., Quinones, J., Fitch, M., et al., (2008). Developing technical expertise in emergency medicine –the role of simulation in procedural skill acquisition. Academic Emergency Medicine, 15, 1046-1057.

Wegner, D. (1989). White Bears and Other Unwanted Thoughts. New York: Penguin. Weisfogel A. & Ross C. Napping: You snooze –you win! CBS News. March 8, 2020. https://www.cbsnews.com/news/napping-you-snooze-you-win/

White, N. (2019). Use of mental imagery to learn CPR skills in pre-registration nurse education. British Journal of Nursing. 28 (7), 468-469.

White T. For weary physicians and nurses, short naps can make a difference. Stanford Report: October 25, 2006. https://news.stanford.edu/news/2006/october25/med-nap-102506.html

Whitelock K & Asken M. ode Calm on the Streets: Mental Toughness Skills for Pre-Hospital Emergency Personnel. 2012; Mechanicsburg, PA: Sunbury Press.

Wilson, T. (2002). Strangers to Ourselves: Discovering the Adaptive Unconscious. Cambridge, MA: Belknap Press of Harvard University.

Wolfson, A. (2005, 4th Ed). Harwood-Nuss' Clinical Practice of Emergency Medicine. Philadelphia: Lippincott, Williams & Wilkins.

Wood, G., & Wilson, M. (2012). Quiet eye training, perceived control and performance under pressure. Psychology of Sport and Exercise. 13 (6), 721-728.

Yoo, S., Gujar, N., Hu, P.et al. (2007). The human emotional brain without sleep – a pre-frontal amygdala disconnect. Current Biology, 17, 877-878.

Zimmerman, L. (2008). Force decision-making. ILEETA Use of Force Journal, 8, (1), 19-21

Notes:

Chapter Quotations:

Introduction: https://www.medelita.com/blog/best-inspirational-nurse-quotes/

Chapter I: https://www.medelita.com/blog/best-inspirational-nurse-quotes/

Chapter II: Scrubs.com

Chapter III: https://www.independenceplus.com/20-quotes-that-inspire-greatness-in-nursing

Chapter IV: Kenny, J.
https://www.nursetheory.com/nursing-quotes/

Chapter V: Scrubs.com

Chapter VI: Juma, N. (2023). Florence Nightingale quotations on life, communication and nursing. Everyday Power: https://everydaypower.com/florence-nightingale-quotes/

Chapter VII: Fountaki, A., et al. (2021). Mater Sociomed.

Chapter VIII: https://www.nursebuff.com/nursing-quotes-2/ Selftalk

Chapter IX: https://www.nursetheory.com/nursing-quotes/

Chapter X: https://www.medelita.com/blog/best-inspirational-nurse-quotes/

Photo Credits

IV 3rd Person: Wavebreakermedia Ltd/ Dreamstime.com

IV 1st Person: La Fabrika Pixel S.T./ Dreamstime.com

About the Authors

Michael J. Asken, MA, PHD.

Mike holds a B.A. degree in Social & Behavioral Sciences from the Johns Hopkins University. He completed his doctoral degree in Clinical Psychology with a minor in Medical Psychology at West Virginia University and received his internship training at the East Orange (New Jersey) Veterans' Administration Hospital. He is a Fellow of the Division of Health Psychology and the Society for Sport, Exercise and Performance Psychology of the American Psychological Association, and the Pennsylvania Psychological Association..

He has been involved in training physicians, intensive care unit nurses, neonatal intensive care unit nurses, nurse anesthetists and enterostomal therapists for over thirty years. He was the psychologist for the Family Practice Residency and Internal Medicine Residency at what is now UPMC Central Pennsylvania Region. He was an adjunct assistant professor of behavioral science at the Milton S. Hershey Medical Center – Pennsylvania State University College of Medicine.

Mike is currently the Senior Organizational Performance Consultant for the Department of Surgery at UPMC Pinnacle Hospitals. There he developed the Surgical MUSE (Mental Underpinnings of Surgical Excellence) initiative and continues to train residents, physicians and nurses in the psychological aspects of surgery and elite performance.

He has been an invited reviewer for Pennsylvania Medicine, the Journal of the American Medical Association, the Western Journal of Medicine, the Sport Psychologist, Adapted Physical Activity Quarterly, Annals of Internal Medicine, the American Surgeon, and the International Journal of Behavioral Medicine and the Journal of Perianesthesia Nursing.

Mike has published articles in the American Journal of Psychiatry, the Journal of Surgical Research, Primary Care, Journal of Family Practice, Pennsylvania Medicine, Journal of Medical Education, Family Medicine, Physician Executive, Journal of the Association of Nurse Anesthetists, Journal of Practical Nursing, Professional Psychology, the International Journal of Sport Psychology, Rehabilitation Psychology, The American Journal Of Surgery, The American Surgeon, Resuscitation, Medical Economics and General Surgery News.

Mike has worked on maximizing performance with athletes at the youth, high school, collegiate and professional levels. He was the sport psychologist for two professional soccer teams, the Hershey Wildcats and the Harrisburg Heat, as well as the semi-pro football team, the Harrisburg Patriots. He is a co-editor of the book: *Sport Psychology: The Psychological Health of the Athlete* and wrote *Dying to Win: Preventing Drug Abuse in Sport.*

While continuing to train residents and physicians, Mike was the psychologist for the Pennsylvania State Police where he was involved with selection and training of Troopers. He functioned as the psychologist for the PSP Special Emergency Response Team, consulting with both tactical operators and crisis negotiators. He was involved with cadet performance issues at the Pennsylvania State Police Academy.

He was an instructor for Top Gun undercover narcotics agent training. He has consulted with and/or provided training for the National Tactical Officers' Association, Eastern States Vice Investigators Association, the International Association of Law Enforcement Firearms Instructors, the New England Crisis Negotiator's Association, the FBI, the Pennsylvania Attorney General's Agents, the United States Postal Inspection

Service, Villanova University Naval ROTC, Navy Special Warfare Group I SEALs, and the U.S. Army War College.

He has written articles for PoliceOne.com., The Crisis Negotiator, The Tactical Edge, Calibre Press Street Survival Newsline, SWAT Digest, Law Officer, The Bulletin of the Pennsylvania Chiefs of Police, the FBI Law Enforcement Bulletin and the FireArms Instructor.

Mike is the author of *MindSighting: Mental Toughness Skills for Police Officers in High Stress Situation* and *Emotional Intel: Mental Toughness Skills for High Stress Crisis Negotiations*. He is co-author with Lt. Colonel Dave Grossman of *Warrior MindSet: Mental Toughness Skills for a Nation' Peacekeepers – Applying Performance Psychology to Combat* and also co-author with Dr. Frank Masur of *Going Deep: Psychoemotional Stress and Survival in an Undercover Police Career*. With Mark Lavallee, MD, he is the co-author of *Rise Above Your Sports Injury*.

Mike is also the author of *Code Calm: Mental Toughness Skills for Medical Emergencies*. With Harold Yang, MD, PhD, he is the co-author of *SIM: The Surgeon's Imagery Mindset*.

Kimberly McMillen, BS, RN, BSN

Kimberly McMillen is a long-term care registered nurse. She began her studies in the healthcare field at Towson University. where she studied health education and health sciences. After graduating, she began her career guiding abused and neglected children in group homes. That led to her seeking her nursing degree, and has been in the profession for over seventeen years. During her career, Kim has provided quality care to patients in major health institutions such as Johns Hopkins Hospital and the University of Maryland health care system. She coordinated the opening and continued managing operation of the Baltimore Field Hospital during the COVID pandemic.

www.ingramcontent.com/pod-product-compliance
Lightning Source LLC
LaVergne TN
LVHW010309070526
838199LV00065B/5496